"Alternative" Healthcare

A Comprehensive Guide

Consumer Health Library®
Series Editor: Stephen Barrett, M.D.
Technical Editor: Manfred Kroger, Ph.D.

"Alternative" Healthcare

A Comprehensive Guide

NATURAL MEDICINE,
"HANDS-ON" HEALING,
SPIRITUALISM, OCCULTISM

AND MUCH MORE

Jack Raso, M.S., R.D.
Edited by Stephen Barrett, M.D.

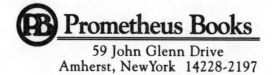

Prometheus Books

59 John Glenn Drive
Amherst, NewYork 14228-2197

Published in 1994 by Prometheus Books.

"Alternative" Healthcare: A Comprehensive Guide. Copyright © 1994 by
Jack Raso. All rights reserved. No part of this publication may be repro-
duced, stored in a retrieval system, or transmitted in any form by any
means, electronic, mechanical, photocopying, recording, or otherwise,
without prior permission of the publisher, except in the case of brief
quotations embodied in critical articles or reviews. Inquiries should be
addressed to Prometheus Books, 59 John Glenn Drive, Buffalo, NY 14228-
2197, 716-691-0133 (FAX: 716-691-0137).

98   97   96   95   94   5   4   3   2   1

Library of Congress Cataloging-in-Publication Data

Raso, Jack
    "Alternative" healthcare : a comprehensive guide / Jack Raso : edited
by Stephen Barrett.
        p.   cm. — (Consumer health library)
    Includes biographical references and index.
    ISBN 0-87975-891-0 (cloth : acid-free paper)
    1. Alternative medicine   I. Barrett, Stephen, 1933–   .
II. Title. III. Series
R733.R37   1994   93-48260
616.85'22--dc29   CIP

For Harry Chung

About the Author

Jack Raso is a registered dietitian who lives in New York City, where he was born and raised. A humanities major from 1972 to 1974, Mr. Raso attended three vocational schools before returning to college in 1981. In 1985, he graduated *summa cum laude* from Pratt Institute in Brooklyn with a B.S. degree in nutrition and dietetics. Later that year, he received a teaching fellowship at Long Island University, where he studied exercise physiology and earned an M.S. degree in health science. Mr. Raso publishes and co-edits *Nutrition Forum*, a newsletter focusing on nutritional and medical fads, fallacies, and controversies. A member of the National Council Against Health Fraud, he also is collaborating on an encyclopedia of "alternative" medicine. His first book, *Mystical Diets: Paranormal, Spiritual, and Occult Nutrition Practices*, was published in 1993 by Prometheus Books.

About the Editor

Stephen Barrett, M.D., a retired psychiatrist, is a nationally renowned author, editor, and consumer advocate. An expert in medical communications, he is medical editor of Prometheus Books and emeritus editor of *Nutrition Forum*. He is a board member of the National Council Against Health Fraud and chairs the council's Task Force on Victim Redress. His thirty-five books include: *The Health Robbers: A Close Look at Quackery in America, Reader's Guide to "Alternative" Health Methods*, and four editions of the college textbook *Consumer Health: A Guide to Intelligent Decisions*. In 1984, he won the FDA Commissioner's Special Citation Award for Public Service. In 1987, he began teaching health education at The Pennsylvania State University.

Contents

Acknowledgments

The author is grateful to the following individuals for their many helpful suggestions during the preparation of the manuscript:

Project manager   Mary A. Read, Assistant Editor, Prometheus Books
Legal advisor   Michael Botts, Esq., Kansas City, Missouri
Technical editor   Manfred Kroger, Ph.D., Professor of Food Science,
                   The Pennsylvania State University
Associate editor   Deborah Anne Barrett, Ph.D. candidate, Stanford
                   University Department of Sociology
Consultant   William T. Jarvis, Ph.D., Professor of Health Promotion
                   and Education, Loma Linda University

The author also thanks Varghese Kodiyan, M.A., M.S.W., C.S.W., Inna Lipnitsky, M.S.L.I.S., Ira Milner, R.D., and Joel Carlinsky for supplying some of the source documents used for this book.

Part I

Spirits in the Material World

1

Mystical Healing: My Odyssey Continues

I use the term "mystical healing" to refer to a vast assortment of approaches whose common denominator is the postulate of "supernatural phenomena." This postulate distinguishes mystical healing not only from scientific medicine but from those modes of "alternative" healthcare that do not posit such phenomena. Several "alternative medicine" proponents I met during the development of this book aptly called my research into mystical practices a journey. However, this investigation was just one part of an odyssey—a continual search for central truths—that began during my adolescence and will probably last until I die. Sometimes it is unpleasant and alienates me from acquaintances and vice versa. Sometimes it bores me. But in 1993 I reached the point of no return.

From Catholicism to *Mystical Diets* and Beyond

My childhood was steeped in religious supernaturalism. I was born in Brooklyn in 1954. Several days later, an Italian-American couple adopted me under circumstances that remain mysterious. My adoptive parents were churchgoing Roman Catholics. During my upbringing and adolescence, I lived in a house where dozens of religious icons were evident: crucifixes and other representations of Jesus Christ, a picture of his "sacred heart," and pictures of his "virgin" mother, sundry saints, and popes. I attended parochial schools from kindergarten through eighth grade. I was an altar boy briefly and a member of the choir for three years. For nine years of intellectual darkness, I regarded nuns, priests,

3

instructors, and the Eucharistic bread of the Mass with awe and accepted without question the teachings of the Catholic catechism. I was so "well behaved" that my class of '68 yearbook said: "If noise were a lumberyard, Jack would be a splinter!"

My religious indoctrination continued, attenuated, throughout four years of diocesan education at Christ the King High School. However, a young priest had planted a seed of doubt when he told my grade-school class that God might not have literally cut a swath through the Red Sea. The progressive modernization of the Roman Catholic Mass weakened its mystical allure for me—and my confidence in Catholicism. But my magical thinking persisted and I became an occultist of sorts.

As my dissatisfaction with Christianity deepened, I turned to other belief systems. For the topic of a paper due in a comparative-religion course, I chose Persian dualism—an ancient tradition positing more than one god. Between 1970 and 1988, I read many uncritical books on such subjects as astrology, the so-called Bermuda triangle, extraterrestrials, Satanism, magic, witchcraft, gods, ghosts, vampires, werewolves, reincarnation, and cultic dietary practices. I submitted to faith healing. I studied the Bible with a Jehovah's Witness who claimed that Armageddon—the end of the world—would begin before I turned twenty-one. I attended meetings of a Japanese Buddhist sect and chanted mindlessly. I ingested nutritional supplements, herbal preparations, and health foods with abandon—despite a half-dozen "side effects." I consulted three "alternative" practitioners. I worked in three health-food stores. And I studied hatha yoga and meditation at the Himalayan Institute of New York.

In 1988, my doubts concerning God and an afterlife peaked after a romance ended in catastrophe. The breakup thrust me into "spiritual bankruptcy." This I sought to remedy through prayers, meditation, creative visualization, crystal therapy, and the contemplative reading of mystical literature—to no avail. On the contrary, I derived strength from the writings of philosophers such as Bertrand Russell and Friedrich Nietzsche, from books upholding atheism and secular humanism, and from rationalistic periodicals such as *Free Inquiry* and *Skeptical Inquirer*.

During my "recovery," I haunted bookstores specializing in mystical and occult literature. My inquisitivenesss attracted opportunities to write about "mystical healing." As a writer, I attended a seminar at the Kushi Institute (the macrobiotic mecca), a Natural Hygiene conference, a conference on the Edgar Cayce approach to healing, a "complementary medicine" symposium, four meetings promoting person-to-person sales of herbal supplements, a lecture by Charlotte Gerson, Newlife Expo '91 ("a symposium of health, environment and spirit"), a nutrition seminar for chiropractors, and a conference on applied kinesiology, ayurveda, and homeopathy. I narrate these experiences in my previous book, *Mystical Diets*, which includes chapters on anthroposophy and theosophy, Gerson therapy, herbalism, nutripathy, nutrition-related products available by mail, and cultic health education.

Mystical Diets emphasizes nutrition cultism or "paranormal nutrition." This book, which overlaps but complements my first, includes an encyclopedic glossary and describes nearly every supernaturalistic health-related method or system currently in use. By "supernaturalistic," I mean involving belief in forces outside of nature—forces that cannot be observed or measured by scientific procedures. My aim from the outset of this project was not to refute mystical healing but to elucidate it from the perspective of a seasoned unbeliever. My descriptions of supernaturalistic methods should help the reader pierce the formidable jargon that proponents delight in using. I adapted these descriptions meticulously from numerous, largely promotional sources: dictionaries, encyclopedias, "monographs," handbooks, magazine articles and ads, directories, book catalogs, course catalogs, pamphlets, circulars, transcripts, and videotapes. I anticipate that this book will be a resource to health professionals and laypeople alike baffled by the maze of "alternative" healthcare and spiritualism. I also hope it will prove an antidote to manuals written by proselytizers. The bibliography comprises most of the books that have contributed to my understanding of mystical healing and supernaturalism.

What I Have Learned

Since I began studying mystical healing in 1989, I have reached four conclusions that strip "alternative" healthcare of much of its allure:

1. Death entails the obliteration of an individual's ability to think, feel, or function purposefully.

2. The word "god" refers to an array of mysterious conceptions—not to any active being.

3. Human beings are not interconnected by supernatural or paranormal forces.

4. "Alternative" healthcare enterprises generally blend selected scientific facts, banalities, and pop-psychological, parapsychological, and magico-religious notions.

In *Fads and Quackery in Healing* (1932), Morris Fishbein, M.D., a fervid opponent of quackery, wrote:

Cult follows cult, and quackery succeeds quackery, frequently with amazing rapidity. Moreover, many cults seem to be definitely confined to small districts and fail to come to light in the available literature on the subject, or even in a careful investigation. Then, too, a single temporarily successful cult . . . gives birth to many offshoots which again propagate more bizarre offspring and unusual hybrids. A complete picture of the farcical scene would require endless research.

So it is today.

"Many Ways to Skin a Cat" (or Fleece a Flock)

The July/August 1992 issue of *Inner Living*, a tabloid-format periodical purporting to be "an inner pivot in the outer world," includes an article titled "Healing Made Simple," in which John Allen states:

> Psychic Healing and the Alternate Methods of Healing (Physical, Mental, or Spiritual) are talked about and given a great deal of publicity today.
> This includes everything from Reiki to Acupressure, from Chakra Healing to Homeopathy. There are many ways to skin a cat. What may work for one person may not for another.
> Once the individual *lingo* is understood for whatever avenue of healing a person looks into—be it chi or energy, meridians or pressure points, eastern or western words—there often can be seen some real basics that most of the disciplines tap into.

Except for Allen's implication of efficacy, I agree. The systems, modalities, and "diagnostic" methods listed below range from the self-evidently and intrinsically supernaturalistic to the quasi-supernaturalistic; from the exclusively health-related to the peripherally or obscurely health-related; and from alternative-medicine "headliners" to "wayside" or highly sectarian approaches. The glossary of this book describes nearly all of these methods and some related concepts. (Foreign terms I did not find in English dictionaries are italicized.)

Absent healing; also called distant healing, distance healing, remote healing, absentee healing, and teleotherapeutics
Actualism; also called agni yoga, fire yoga, and lightwork. Includes actualism bodywork
Acupressure; also called *G-jo*. Includes acu-ball pressure self-treatment **and** *do-in* (also spelled "dao-in"; also called Taoist yoga)
Acupuncture; also called acupuncture therapy. Includes electroacupuncture (also called electrical acupuncture)

Acupuncture, homuncular. Includes auriculotherapy (also called auricular therapy, auricular acupuncture, and ear acupuncture) and reflexotherapy

Acuscope therapy; also called electro-acuscope therapy

Acu-yoga

African holistic health

Agni dhatu; also called *agni dhatu* therapy and *samadhi* yoga

Aikido

Alchemical hypnotherapy; also called alchemical work

Alexander technique; also called the Alexander method

Alternative twelve steps

Amma therapy®

Amulet healing

Angelic healing

Annette Martin training

Anthroposophical medicine; also called anthroposophically-extended medicine. Includes therapeutic eurythmy (also spelled "eurhythmy"; also called curative eurythmy)

Applied kinesiology (AK); also called kinesiology. Includes the LePore technique

Archetypal psychology

Aroma behavior conditioning (ABC)

Aromatherapy

Aromics™

Astanga yoga; also spelled "ashtanga"; also called raja yoga

Astara's healing science

Aston-patterning®

Astrologic medicine; also called astral healing, astrological healing, astromedicine, and medical astrology

Astrology, psychological; also called astro-psychology

Attunement

Aura balancing; also called auric healing, aura healing, aura cleansing, and aura clearing. Includes auric massage technique

Aurasomatherapy

Auricular reflexology

AVATAR

"Awakened Life" program

Ayurveda; also called ayurvedic medicine, ayurvedic healing, Vedic medicine, and ayurvedism. Includes marma therapy (also called ayurvedic massage and ayurvedic lymphatic massage)

Bach flower therapy

Baguazhang; also called *pa kua chang* and circle walking

Balance therapy

Behavioral kinesiology (BK)

Biblical counseling; also called nouthetic counseling
Bindegewebsmassage; also called the bindegewebsmassage system
Bio-chromatic chakra alignment
Biodynamic massage
Bioenergetics, encompassing bioenergetic analysis and bioenergetic therapy
Bioenergy; also called bioenergy healing
Biomagnetics; also called biomagnetic medicine
Bioplasmic healing
Biorhythm(s)
Biosonics
Body harmony
Body integration
Bodymind centering
Bodywork plus
Bodywork tantra, encompassing watsu, tantsu, and co-centering
BRETH ("Breath Releasing Energy for Transformation and Healing" or "Breath
    Releasing Energy for Transformation and Happiness")
Bubble of light technique; also called bubble of light meditation
Buddhism, Esoteric

Cayce approach to health and healing. Includes Cayce/Reilly massage
Cellular theta breath; also called cellular theta breath technique
Chakra energy massage
Chakra healing; also called chakra therapy, chakra balancing, chakra energy
    balancing, and chakra work. Includes chakra breathing and chakra innertuning
    therapy
Chan Mi gong
Channeling; also called mediumship. Includes trance channeling
Chen-chiou therapy
Chi kung meditation(s)
Chinese hand analysis
Chinese Qigong massage, including amma (also called *anma* and *pu tong an mo*),
    tui na (also called *tui na an mo*), and *dian xue* (also called *dian xue an mo*)
Chinese system of food cures
Chirognomy; also spelled "cheirognomy"
Chiropractic, fundamentalist
Christian meditation (C.M.)
Clairvoyant diagnosis; also called psychic diagnosis
Color breathing
Color meditation (CM); also called color magick
Color psychology
Color synergy
Color therapy; also called chromotherapy, color healing, and chromopathy.
    Includes color projection

Concept-therapy®; also called concept-therapy technique. Comprises suggestive
therapy (also called suggestive therapy work and suggestive therapeutics) and
suggestive therapy zone procedure (also called zone therapy diagnosis, health
zone analysis, concept-therapy adjusting technique, and zone testing)
Contact healing; also called the laying on of hands
Core energetics; also called core energetic therapy
Cosmic energy *chi kung*; also called cosmic healing *chi kung* and cosmic *chi kung*.
Cosmic vibrational healing
A Course in Miracles
Craniosacral therapy; also called cranial technique, cranial osteopathy, craniopathy,
craniosacral balancing, craniosacral work, and cranial work
Creative visualization (see Glossary for related terms)
Crystal therapy; also called crystal healing, crystal work, and crystal therapeutics
Cupping, including *bu-hang*
Cymatics; also called cymatic medicine and cymatic therapy

Dayan Qigong; also called wild goose breathing exercise
de la Warr system
Diamond approach; also called the Diamond approach to inner realization
Diamond method
Dianetics
Dreamwork; also called dreamworking

EAV (electroacupuncture according to Voll)
Eighteen lohan tiger/dragon Qigong
Electrodiagnosis; also called electrodermal screening and bioelectric testing
Electro-homeopathy
Electromagnetic healing
Electromedicine
EmBodyment
Empyrean® rebirthing
Endo-nasal therapy
Energy balancing
Enneagram system; also called enneagram
Equestrian transformational expression; also called horseback to heaven
Er Mei Qigong; also called *Er Mei*
Esalen massage
Esoteric healing; also called the seven ray techniques
Etheric surgery
Eutony; also called eutony therapy and the Gerda Alexander method
Exorcism, including depossession (also called releasement)

Face modelling
Facial rejuvenation-Burnham system®

Faith healing, including Christian healing (such as Christian evangelical healing
    and Christian Science)
Ferreri technique
Firewalking
Flower essence therapy
Foot analysis; also called the Grinberg method

Gem therapy
Gerson therapy; also called Gerson treatment, the Gerson method, and Gerson
    dietary regime (GDR)
Graphochromopathy
Graphology, medical; also called grapho-diagnostics
Graphotherapy

Hakomi; also called the hakomi method, hakomi therapy, and hakomi body-
    centered psychotherapy
Harmonics
Hatha yoga
Healing *tao*; also called the healing *tao* system, the international healing *tao*
    system, and healing *tao* warm current meditation. Includes bone marrow *nei
    kung* (also called iron shirt *chi kung* III), *chi nei tsang* (also called Taoist *chi nei
    tsang*, Taoist healing light technique, internal organ *chi* massage, organ *chi*
    transformation massage, and organ *chi* transformation and healing light
    massage), *chi* self-massage (also called *tao* rejuvenation-*chi* self-massage),
    fusion meditations, healing light kung fu (also called healing hands kung fu),
    healing love (also called healing love meditation and "seminal and ovarian kung
    fu"), inner smile, iron shirt *chi kung*, microcosmic orbit meditation, the six
    healing sounds, and Taoist five element nutrition (also called Taoist healing
    diet)
Hellerwork
Hemi-sync™
Hippocrates health program, including the Hippocrates diet (also called living
    foods lifestyle)
Holistic dentistry
Holistic gynecology
Holistic nursing
Holistic palpate energy therapy
Holistic reiki
Holotropic breathwork™; also called holotropic therapy, holotropic breath therapy,
    holonomic breathwork, holonomic therapy, and Grof breathwork
Homeoacupuncture
Homeopathy; also called homeopathic medicine and homeotherapeutics
Homeovitics
Human energetic assessment and restorative technic (HEART)

Hydrochromopathy
Hydropathy; also called water cure
Hypnoaesthetics™

Identity process
Imagineering
Ingham technique; also called the Ingham method
Inner bonding
Inner child therapy; also called inner child work
Inner self healing process
Integral counseling psychology
Integrative acupressure
Integrative therapy
Interactive guided imagery℠
Iridology; also called iridiagnosis and irido-diagnosis
Iyengar yoga; also called Iyengar style yoga

Jin shinn; also spelled "jin shin." Includes *jin shin jyutsu* (also spelled "jitsu") and
   jin shin do® (also called jin shin do® bodymind acupressure™)
Josephing
Jungian psychology

Kahuna healing (including lomi-lomi) and other forms of shamanism (also called
   shamanic healing and shamanistic medicine)
Ki breathing
Ki-shiatsu®/oriental bodywork; also called ki-shiatsu/oriental bodywork therapy
   and shiatsu oriental bodywork
Kirlian diagnosis (also called Kirlian technique) and other forms of aura analysis
   (also called aura reading)
Kneipping; also called Kneipp cure, Kneipp therapies, and *Kneipptherapie*
Kofutu system of spiritual healing and development, including kofutu touch
   healing and kofutu absent healing
Kripalu bodywork
Kripalu yoga
Kriya yoga
Kulkarni naturopathy
Kum nye; also called *kum nye* relaxation

Lama yoga
Lane system of multilayer bioenergy analysis and nutrition; also called the Lane
   system of 3-dimensional bioenergy analysis and nutritional healing
L'Chaim yoga
Lemonade diet; also called the master cleanser and lemon cleansing
LeShan psychic training

Life energy analysis
Life force balancing
Life impressions bodywork
Light work

Macrobiotics
Magical diet(s)
Magical herbalism
Magnet therapy; also called magnetic therapy, magnetotherapy, magnetic energy
    therapy, magnetic healing, biomagnetics, biomagnetism, biomagnetic therapy,
    and electro-biomagnetics. Includes imaginetics
Magnetic healing
Mahikari
Makko-ho
Manifesting; also called manifestation and conscious manifestation
Manual organ stimulation therapy (MOST)
MariEL
Medipatch™ healthcare system; also called the Medipatch™ system.
Mesmerism; also called magnetic healing
Metamorphic technique; also called metamorphosis (originally called prenatal
    therapy)
Middle pillar meditation; also called middle pillar technique
Morter HealthSystem, including B.E.S.T. (bio energetic synchronization technique)
    and Baby B.E.S.T.
Moxibustion, including moxabustion
Mucusless diet healing system

Natural Hygiene
Nature cure; also called nature care
Naturopathy; also called naturopathic medicine and naturology
NETWORK
Neural organization technique (NOT)
New age shiatsu
Nichiren Buddhism; also called Nichiren Soshu (also spelled "Shoshu") and
    Nichirenism
Numbers diet™ (Jean Simpson's numbers diet)
Numerology
Nutripathy
Nutritional herbology

Ohashiatsu®
Oki-do
OMEGA

Organic process therapy (OPT)
Organismic psychotherapy
Orgone therapy; also called medical orgonomy and orgonomic medicine
Orionic healing system
Ortho-bionomy™
Osteopuncture

Palmistry, medical. Includes Chinese hand analysis
Past-life therapy; also called past lives therapy, regression therapy, past-life
    regression therapy, and transformational therapy
Pathwork
Pealeism
Phoenix rising yoga therapy
Phrenology; also called head-reading
Phreno-mesmerism; also called phreno-magnetism and phrenopathy
Physiognomy
Pigeon remedy; also called pigeon therapy
Plant alchemy; also called spagyrics
Polarity balancing; also called polarity therapy, polarity, polarity wellness®,
    polarity energy balancing, polarity energy balancing system, polarity system,
    and polarity energy healing
Polarity testing
Postural integration
Prakrtika cikitsa; also called naturopathy
Pranic healing; also called bioplasmic healing and radiatory healing. Includes
    invocative pranic healing, color pranic healing, dis®tant pranic healing, and
    pranic psychotherapy
Prayer; also called metaphysical healing. Includes petitionary prayer (personal and
    intercessory)
Primal therapy
Process psychology; also called process oriented psychology
Progression/regression therapy
Psionic medicine; also called psionics
Psychic dentistry
Psychic healing; also called *psi* healing and psychic therapy
Psychic surgery
"Psychology of evil"
Psychometric analysis (short for "psychometric analysis of human character and
    mentality")
Psychometry; also called object reading
Psycho-neuro integration (PNI); also called psychic healing
Psycho-regression
Psychospiritual holistic healing

Psychospiritual therapy
Psychosynthesis; also called psychosynthesis therapy
Pyramid power; also called pyramid energy

Qigong; also spelled "chi gong," "chi gung," and "chi kung"; also called internal
    Qigong. Includes Taoist Qigong (Daoist *chi kung*)
Qi gong meridian therapy
Qigong therapy; also called medical Qigong, *Qi* healing, external *Qi* healing,
    Qigong healing, external Qigong healing, *buqi*, *buqi* therapy, *Qi an mo*, *Qi*
    massage, *wai Qi liao fa*, and *wai Qi zhi liao*

Radiance breathwork
Radiance movement therapy
Radiance prenatal process
Radiesthesia; also called medical radiesthesia and medical dowsing. Includes
    pendular diagnosis (also called radiesthetic diagnosis) and telediagnosis (also
    called distant biological detection)
Radionics; also called psionics. Encompasses radionic diagnosis (also called
    radionic analysis), radionic photography, and radionic therapy (also called
    radionic healing and radionic treatment)
Radix; also called neo-Reichian therapy
Ray methods of healing
Rainbow diet (Dr. Gabriel Cousens's rainbow diet)
Rebirthing; also called conscious breathing, conscious connected breathing,
    circular breathing, free breathing, and vivation
Reflexology, including ear, hand, foot, and body reflexology
Reichian therapy; also called Reichian massage, Reichian bodywork therapy, and
    psychiatric orgone therapy. Called vegetal therapy in Europe
Reiki; also called the Usui system of natural healing, Usui *shiko ryoho*, Usui *shiki
    ryoho*, reiki healing, and reiki therapy; formerly called leiki. Includes the
    radiance technique® (also called real reiki®)
Reiki plus®; also called the reiki plus system of natural healing. Encompasses
    PSEBSM, psycho-therapeutic reikiSM, and spinal attunementSM technique
Remote diagnosis
Rhythmajik
Rolfing®; also called structural integration and structural processing
Rubenfeld synergy® method; also called Rubenfeld synergy

Schuessler (also spelled "Schussler") biochemic system of medicine; also called
    biochemic system of medicine, biochemic medicine, and tissue salts therapy
Sclerology
Scrying; also called crystal gazing, crystal ball, and crystalomancy
Seichim
Seichim reiki

Seiki-jutsu
Self-applied health enhancement methods (SAHEM)
Self-healing; also called direct healing
Shiatsu; also spelled "shiatzu" and "schiatsu"; also called shiatsu therapy. Includes
    shiatsu massage, acupressure, and Zen shiatsu
Siddha; also called Siddha medicine
Silva mind control; also called the Silva mind control system and the Silva method
Simonton method
Soaring crane Qigong; also called crane style *chi gong*
Sotai; also called sotai therapy and sotai treatment
Soul part integration
Soul retrieval
Spinal balancing
Spirit healing; also called spiritual healing
Spirit surgery
Spiritual psychology
Sufi healing
Synergy hypnosis
Systematic nutritional muscle testing (SNMT)

Tai chi; also spelled "tai ji"; also called tai chi chuan (*tai ji chuan, tai ji quan*).
    Includes Chen style
Tanden breathing
Tantra
Theotherapy
Therapeutic touch and noncontact therapeutic touch
Tibetan medicine; also called *Emchi*. Includes Tibetan pulsing (also called Tibetan
    pulsing healing)
Toning
Touch for Health
Trager; also called the Trager approach, Tragerwork, Tragering, and Trager
    psychophysical integration®
Trager mentastics; also called mentastics®
Transcendental meditation (TM) and TM-Sidhi
"Transformation" program
Transformational bodywork
Transpersonal hypnotherapy
Transpersonal psychology; also called transpersonal counseling
Triggers™ mind programming system; also called triggers
Twelve steps

Unani; also called Unani medicine and *Unani tibb*
Urine therapy; also called uropathy, auto-urine-therapy, *amaroli,* and *shivambu*
    kalpa

Vita flex; also called the reflex system
Viviano method

Warriorobics
White tantra
Whole person bodywork
Wise woman healing; also called wisewoman healing ways and wisewoman ways
Witchcraft

Yantra yoga; also called Tibetan yantra yoga
Yoga of perfect sight
Yoga therapy

Zarlen therapy
Zen Alexander technique
Zen-touch™
Zone therapy; also called reflex zone therapy

The next chapter examines the philosophic roots of "alternative" healthcare and distinguishes between science and pseudoscience. Chapter 3 defines the supernaturalistic theories that underlie mystical healing and then focuses on the hypothetical "life force." Chapter 4 illustrates how born-again "medicine" has flourished in pop culture. Parts II, III, and IV deal with "spiritual healing" (e.g., yoga), "natural healing" (e.g., naturopathy), and "hands-on healing" (e.g., reflexology), respectively. Part IV features accounts of my visits to practitioners.

2

Pillars of Unreason

In the Winter 1990 issue of *Skeptical Inquirer*, Erik Strommen wrote: "Alternative health philosophies, taken as a group, seem a veritable Tower of Babel. They represent a confusing democracy of beliefs, jargon, and ritual that together comprise an indistinct, overlapping collection of ideas." Terms such as "alternative," "complementary," "extentional," "fringe," "holistic," "innovative," "mind/body," "nontraditional," "unconventional," and "unorthodox" merely convey that "alternative" healthcare is somehow different from regular healthcare.

What characteristics distinguish the so-called alternatives to conventional medicine? This chapter describes the two theories that constitute the faulty bedrock of "alternative" healthcare and its many magico-religious ideas and precepts. I also convey why mystical methods retain their appeal despite the proliferation of science.

Empiricism and Skepticism Gone Amok

"Alternative" healthcare ultimately stands, shiftily, on two philosophic pillars: *unscientific empiricism* and *universal skepticism*. Moderate empiricism (based on meticulous observation) and qualified skepticism (whereby methodical doubt leads to constructive criticism) are elements of the scientific method. However, both extreme empiricism and total skepticism are akin to mysticism—the stuff of Hinduism and ayurveda.

Unscientific empiricism esteems knowledge derived from experience—trial and error—but devalues knowledge gained by analysis and the systematic organization of information. Medical empirics use experience as a substitute for

17

scientific knowledge in selecting or improvising therapies. They cite scientific studies only when they appear to support what they already "know" from personal observation. They reject scientific testing of their opinions and maintain that their own clinical observations are more valuable than stringently controlled, peer-reviewed experiments. A diehard empiric might even assert, for example, that dreaming or hallucinating about doing something and actually doing it are equivalent experiences. Such notions have receptive audiences in the world of mystical healing.

Viennese pharmacist and ayurveda proponent Birgit Heyn exalts empiricism in *Ayurveda: The Indian Art of Natural Medicine and Life Extension* (1990):

> This demand for proof, understandable and desirable though it may be, does become a problem if it is made the sole criterion; for the implied doubt as to the value of direct perception through the senses and the refusal to use intuition, our "sixth" sense, is abandonment of a vital feature of Ayurveda. Science and technology should be our tools, not replacements for personal knowing and feeling.

Heyn seems to regard science as useful only to the extent that it confirms what individuals surmise, intuit, or want to believe.

In *The Magical Staff: The Vitalist Tradition in Western Medicine* (1992), homeopathy proponent Matthew Wood goes further:

> Since human beings are deeply affected by subjective, spiritual, and even supernatural events, it is impossible to create an adequate system of healing for them which does not include this side of their being. . . .
> If medicine is to address the patient in a realistic manner it is going to have to make peace with the hidden side of humanity. How is this to be done? How can people used to mistrusting their own instincts learn to discern and judge from a subjective standpoint?. . .
> The way to learn to perceive in this fashion is to learn to trust "what feels right." No one can learn to use this kind of knowledge by copying other people. Each person works out what is right for him or her self.
> This procedure will always give results which are similar to . . . a bunch of themes that seem to disagree in important ways, but which, on deeper reflection, are found to support each other. The subjective world is like that. . . .
> If medicine is to address the patient in a way which is realistic, it must encompass our true nature. It must include the spirit, the life force, and the wisdom of nature in its view. Rather than beginning with the body and excluding all other phenomena as subjective and unreliable, medicine must begin at the central point, the magical staff.

In *Space, Time, and Medicine* (1985), Larry Dossey, M.D., recounts a case in which a patient's supernatural beliefs were paramount. The hospitalized patient, an elderly man who appeared to be dying without any evident disease, claimed he was the victim of a shaman's evil spell. Dossey and a fellow intern named Jim developed a "de-hexing" ceremony to "cure" the patient. They covertly enacted this ceremony in an examination room around midnight on a weekend. Dossey describes it:

> I was witnessing an archetypal struggle—one shaman battling another . . . .
>
> Jim produced from his pocket a pair of stainless steel surgical scissors he had "borrowed" for the occasion. In the faint blue light they gleamed as he moved toward the old man, who sat transfixed in his wheelchair, following every one of Jim's slow, deliberate moves. He walked to the wheelchair, raised the scissors, and grasping a lock of gray hair with his other hand began slowly to cut.
>
> The old man seemed by then to have stopped breathing. With the lock of hair in his left hand Jim slowly retreated to the desk top, appearing massive as he stood over the dancing flame. Then he looked squarely at his rigid, wasted patient and said slowly in a calm, deep voice, "As the fire burns your hair, the hex in your body is destroyed." He lowered his hand, allowing the hair to fall into the flame. Then he added the whimsical caution, "But if you reveal this ceremony to anyone, the hex will return immediately, stronger than before!" (I was grateful that Jim was a shaman who was aware of potential professional humiliation!)

Although this case is presented as a "cure," questions remain. Did Dossey and his colleague consider the emotions that caused the man's problem or that his belief system was pathological? Did they consider the possible consequences of reinforcing magical beliefs? Wouldn't such treatment leave the patient vulnerable to further "hexes" or—worse—encourage him to seek shamanic care for a serious illness that only scientific medicine can remedy?

Universal skepticism is more insidious and elusive than empiricism. In its extreme form, it holds that humans cannot know anything—that truth and falsity are indistinguishable. This is absurd because it entails that humans cannot know whether the standpoint itself is true. In its other main form, universal skepticism holds that humans can never be *certain* about anything. This standpoint is likewise absurd because it casts doubt on itself.

Healthy skepticism—the tendency to disbelieve—is often a commendable impetus to learning (represented by the maxim "Look before you leap"). But mystical "skeptics" hold that attempts to verify claims or justify actions are futile because everything is open to doubt or interpretation. Thus in "alterna-

_" healthcare, mystical practitioners and their patients are the arbiters of treatment efficacy and put whatever appeals to them on a therapeutic pedestal.

Whereas modern medicine relies on science, "alternative" healthcare is a rampart for religious principles and pseudoscience.

The Influence of Religion

Faith—steadfast belief without logical proof or material evidence, or belief contrary to evidence—is one of the world's most time-honored attitudes. It is supposedly the key to everlasting bliss, knowledge, and health. In the form of religion, it is a major link with the distant past and its magical follies. The healing-faith connection has ancient roots; the first "doctors" were shamans, and religion and medicine have been entangled throughout history.

Faith is also a central Christian virtue—a prerequisite for heaven. Near the turn of the first century C.E., Tertullian, the first Christian theologian to write in Latin, declared: "I believe because it is absurd." Augustine, another church father, pronounced faith the path to knowledge. The "primacy of faith" doctrine holds that faith precedes reason—that logic, science, knowledge, and the very existence of the material world stem from faith. In defense of this dogma, some religionists employ variations of universal skepticism—the "conviction" (with a built-in refutation) that humans cannot know (or pin down) anything. Consider, for example, the old saying "God only knows." But universal skepticism vindicates nothing. Rather, it engenders chaos—which delusional skeptics mistake for profundity.

"Alternative" healthcare cradles the main objects of faith: God and an afterlife. This relationship between healing and supernatural beliefs is prevalent in each of its branches: "spiritual healing," "natural healing," and bodywork. In the province of "spiritual healing," unbelievers purportedly risk watering down the healing process.

Paul Johannes Tillich (1886–1965), an influential Protestant theologian, defined religion—symbolized by God—as humankind's ultimate concern. He promoted a peaceful separation of philosophy (critical inquiry) and religion (faith). In the essay "Religion and Health," Tillich equated "the cosmic disease" with "cosmic guilt," healers with saviors, and "cosmic healing" with salvation. He stated that the priest is "always and essentially" a medicine man. "He who has the healing power," he continued, "does not have it for himself, but from a special transmission of the universal healing power unto him. The healing power is rooted in the divine realm." According to Tillich, union with divine beings is the means of healing or salvation.

More recently, in *Medicine and Religion: Strategies of Care* (1980), several contributors argued for the inclusion of religious studies in medical education. The editor, Donald W. Shriver, Jr., Ph.D., a pastor and theologian, wrote:

> Stereotypically considered, religion is placed in opposition to the major "virtues" of modern society: faith versus scientific rigor; salvation in another world versus technological solutions to human problems; adherence to antique ideas versus progress and improvement. Over against this stereotype stand the experience and the claims of our group's medical practitioners, who insist that they see the influence of religion in their patients, in themselves, and in their colleagues.

In his back-matter biography, Shriver reported "a mounting accumulation of personal complaints about medicine and its professionalization." For instance, he was "loath to remember" the "pseudo-authority and moral cynicism" of his wife's gynecologist. Two other contributors proposed a sample academic program with courses covering: "the healer as a religious figure," "religious healing" as "the alternative to 'scientific' medicine," the "religious significance" of "laetrile and other nonscientific remedies," and relationships between psychiatric terms and religious themes.

Science versus Pseudoscience

Science is a continuous, complex process whose basic purposes are to identify phenomena and to predict events. It is not a collection of facts but a method of reasoning. Its current of interdependent activities includes: (1) observing and describing phenomena and forming general conclusions about them (empiricism); (2) integrating new data into a systematically organized body of related observations that have been confirmed; (3) formulating testable hypotheses based on the results of this integration; (4) testing the hypotheses under stringently controlled, repeatable conditions; (5) observing results, recording them unambiguously, and interpreting them clearly; and (6) actively seeking criticism (reasonable skepticism) from others engaged in science.

This process—known as the scientific method—has produced knowledge that contradicts cherished articles of faith. But faith is a law unto itself. In *The Atheist Debater's Handbook* (1983), B.C. Johnson wrote:

> Science searches for *correct* explanations and does not settle for known or adequate ones. If science had been content to explain every puzzling phenomenon by saying that God caused it, there would have been no scientific progress whatsoever. Just imagine the knowledge science would have accumulated by now if it had taken this route. All

scientific knowledge would consist of one thing: God. No electrons, atoms or molecules would be invoked as explanations. What causes fire to burn? God. What causes lightning? God. What causes rain? God. The success of science in developing correct explanations has been based solely on its refusal to take the easy way out and proclaim God as the explanation.

"Alternative" healthcare does not merely take such an "easy way out." It often attempts to misrepresent its supernaturalistic basis by embroidering it with scientific and pseudoscientific jargon. Thus it maintains a facade of secularity and respectability.

Daisie Radner and Michael Radner describe the characteristics of pseudo-science in *Science and Unreason* (1982). These include: (1) anachronistic thinking—dusting off and championing a refuted theory because of its moral appeal; (2) mystery-seeking—making the search for anomalies and enigmas one's primary aim; (3) mythmongering—making myths the starting-point for research or invoking them to promote a theory; (4) a lopsided approach to evidence—accepting unreliable (unconfirmed) findings that support a favored theory; (5) construction of hypotheses that preclude disproof—stating an argument in a way that negates testing; (6) false comparison—outfitting unscientific practices with the accouterments of science; (7) "literary criticism" of the scientific literature—taking the entire body of scientific literature as one's field of study, and picking and choosing statements therein to support a theory; and (8) refusal to revise a theory in response to legitimate criticism.

When science is made subservient to empiricism and universal skepticism, supernaturalism is enthroned. Many gurus, faithmongers, quacks, and conventional religionists would make supernaturalism the quintessence of healthcare. But the mingling of religion and healthcare (scientific or unscientific) opens the door to all manner of mumbo-jumbo and whimsicality. The following chapter describes some of the supernaturalistic theories to which mystical "healers" give their allegiance.

3

Carnival of Souls

Alleged supernatural beings and forces are, by definition, mysterious—and probably inherently incomprehensible, since beings and forces are explicitly definable only in naturalistic terms. The keystone of "alternative" healthcare is a supposed semiautonomy of the body and mind—or of the body, mind, and spirit. Proponents tend to blur the distinction between mind and spirit (soul). Yet an understanding of this distinction is crucial to the unraveling of many "alternative" approaches.

In scientific healthcare, the word "mind" refers basically to sequences of thoughts and sensations—a process that occurs continuously until death. The mind is not a material (physical) thing but a concept representing the multitudinous physiologic (cellular-level) events that constitute thinking. The spirit (soul) likewise is not a material thing, but, unlike the mind, it has no basis in physiology.

Naturalism versus Supernaturalism

Naturalism—the basis of science—holds that the universe (natural world) is all that exists and that all phenomena are explainable, at least in principle, without recourse to supernatural ideas. Supernaturalism—its antithesis—declares that there are powers outside the natural world and that those powers at least occasionally affect the courses of events. In *Atheism: The Case Against God* (1989), George H. Smith wrote: "The controversy between naturalism and supernaturalism is not a contest between two rival modes of explanation; it is

23

not a matter of which provides a better explanation. Rather, it is an issue of explanation versus no explanation whatsoever."

The following ten supernaturalistic theories are relevant to "alternative" healthcare:

- *Idealism (mentalism or immaterialism):* Matter does not exist; mind or spirit is the only reality.

- *Soul/body dualism:* Human beings consist of a body and a soul, which are separable; thinking and volition take place in the soul.

- *Mind/body dualism:* Mind and body are disparate and separable.

- *Mind/body interactionism:* Mind and body are disparate entities that affect each other.

- *Animism (panpsychism):* Everything in the universe possesses a mind or soul in varying degrees.

- *Mind-stuff theory:* "Psychic material" is present in varying amounts in everything down to the smallest particle.

- *Theism:* (1) There is a perfect, eternal, almighty, omniscient, benevolent being who created and rules the universe, i.e., God (monotheism); or (2) there are several or many supernatural beings who control nature (polytheism); or (3) there is a supernatural being who created but completely transcends the universe; humanity's highest duty is to follow this being's immutable universal laws (deism).

- *Pantheism:* "God" and "nature" are synonymous. (Pantheism, which has an affinity with Eastern mysticism, is both naturalistic and trivial unless the believer ascribes supernatural phenomena or a morality to "nature." Unnecessary capitalization of the word "nature" usually indicates supernaturalistic pantheism.)

- *Mysticism:* All conclusions, beliefs, and opinions based on analysis, deduction, and/or common experience are illusory. True knowledge is attainable only through contemplative or intuitive union (or near-union) with God, a "higher reality," or the universe, but such knowledge is indescribable. Intense feeling marks this union or near-union.

- *Vitalism:* An invisible, intangible, unique form of energy is responsible for all the activities of a living organism and (according to some vitalists) can exist independently of the organism.

Vitalism is the ruling principle of "alternative" healthcare. Its most influential form in the United States is the doctrine of salvation, which holds that: (1) humans have—or are—souls; (2) every soul continues to exist despite bodily death; and (3) at death, souls go to heaven or hell. Many mystical philosophers equate the mind with the soul and liken the body to a temporary prison. Some vitalists assert that food can be "dead" or "living" and that "live" foods contain a dormant or primitive "life force" that humans can assimilate.

Vitalism's popularity stems from its compatibility with everyday religious notions, the desire to believe that humankind is more than just another item of matter, and, above all, the universal hope that nonphysical human characteristics will outlast the human body in a coherent form and amount to "life after death." In the realms of religion and pseudomedicine, vitalism and theism are potent bedfellows. For example, *The Art of True Healing* (1991) states: "The force of life is infinite; we are saturated, permeated through and through with this spiritual force, this energy. It constitutes our higher self, it is our link with Godhead, it is God within us."

Mysticism—second only to vitalism in the realm of "alternative" medicine—posits "realities" not apprehensible by the intellect but approachable through subjective, extrasensory experience. Critics of this belief have characterized mystics as obstinate malcontents who deny the world in order to find reality. According to mysticism, the "vital force" is not part of human beings; rather, humans are manifestations of a divine and infinite "Life." The principal form of mysticism in "alternative" healthcare is Hindu mysticism—the worldview of yoga and ayurveda. Hindu mysticism holds that death is an illusion and that people can escape it and "relapse" into "Immortal Vitality" by abolishing their individuality (see Chapter 5).

Spirits in the Material World

Vitalism hinges on the existence of a nonmaterial, divine, or personalized form of energy. Yet it is a principle of physics that matter and energy are interconvertible—two forms of the same thing. Einstein formulated this axiom as $E = mc^2$—the energy of an object equals its mass times the square of the speed of light.

Thus: (1) energy *must* be a form of matter and be *devoid* of personality, and (2) nonmaterial things can "exist" only as thoughts and are not measurable. Medical vitalists ignore this first fact but trumpet the second as though it supports their beliefs. The generic terms they use for their pseudo-energy include: vital force *(force vitale)*, vital energy, inner vital energy, vital cosmic force, vital energy force, vital element, vital principle, vital spirit, vital life spirit, vital magnetism, vitalistic principle, life force, life power, universal life force, cosmic life force, vital life force, vital life force energy, life energy, universal life energy, cosmic life energy, universal life force energy, internal energy, nerve force, nerve energy, personal energy, subtle energy, vitality energy, energy of being, the force of life, and élan vital. In addition to these synonyms, there are dozens of terms for the same idea that carry the flavor of particular belief systems. These include: animal magnetism (mesmerism), *chi* or *Qi* (ancient Chinese tradition), etheronic force (Edgar Cayce), innate intelligence or Innate (Daniel David Palmer, the founder of chiropractic), *ki* (Japanese tradition, Shinto), mana (ancient Hawaiian tradition, Huna), *prana* (Hinduism), reiki (Usui system), soul or spirit (Christianity), and *vis medicatrix naturae* (naturopathy).

Other terms for alleged forms of energy relevant to "alternative" healthcare include: bio-current, bioenergy, biomagnetic waves, bioplasma (bioplasmic energy or psychotronic energy), entelechy, essence, kundalini (Shakti), life-fields (L-fields, electrodynamic fields, or bioelectric fields), M-fields, morphogenic fields (morphogenetic fields, morphic fields, or morphic resonance), odic force (od or odyle), orgone (orgone energy or bions), paraelectricity, psi-fields, psi plasma, psychic energy (psychic force), *seiki*, tachyon energy (tachyon field energy), *vis formativa*, and zero-point energy (virtual energy). In *Reiki: Universal Life Energy* (1988), "spiritual healers" Bodo J. Baginski and Shalila Sharamon state that *"ki"* and twenty-eight other terms probably refer to "one and the same basic energy, although the extent to which they are applied and the theories concerning them differ greatly." In *The Encyclopedia of Alternative Health Care* (1989), "holistic health educator" Kristin Gottschalk Olsen, M.S., equates the "life force" or "vital force" with *chi, ki, prana*, electromagnetism, and "the Force" in the movie "Star Wars." But in the Winter 1993 issue of *Noetic Sciences Review*, another proponent, biophysicist Beverly Rubik, states:

> Science does not have a good hold on the concept of subtle life energies—such as ch'i, prana, orgone energy, entelechy or vital force. The phenomenon has been given many names throughout history. I would certainly not equate it with electromagnetism at this point.

Energy Detection?

Although they characterize it diversely, proponents of "alternative" medicine agree that the "vital force" is detectable—*subjectively*. In *Essence: The Diamond Approach to Inner Realization* (1986), A.H. Almaas states that people seldom recognize the "vital force" because it "does not fall within those usual categories of thought, emotion, and physical sensation." "The difficulty," he continues, "is that the reality that is sought is in a form that is not expected. The person might even be looking it in the face but not realize it is what he is looking for." According to Almaas, the "vital force"—which he calls "essence"—"is within us just as space is within us," but "it is not empty the way physical space is." "It has," he explains, "a substantiality similar to the physical body but in a different dimension." Almaas states that essence "is not a state of mind but . . . actual and palpable." Yet he claims that people can perceive or experience it directly "when there is a strong energetic discharge as in deep emotion."

Such pompous gobbledygook is typical of vitalistic apologists. In *The Energy Within* (1992), Richard M. Chin, a martial artist and "doctor of Oriental medicine," asserts that one can "actually *feel*" the vital force if one suspends disbelief "long enough to begin the work to find it." Apparently, the "right" frame of mind makes "perception" of the so-called vital force unavoidable.

In *Ageless Body, Timeless Mind: The Quantum Alternative To Growing Old* (1993), Deepak Chopra describes *prana* as "the subtlest form of biological energy" and as "intelligence and consciousness, the two vital ingredients that animate physical matter." He states:

> The experience of Prana can be had in many ways: When you are flushed with sudden energy, feel the inrush of sudden alertness and clarity, or simply perceive that you are "in the flow," your attention has been drawn to Prana. Some people sense it as a streaming or buzzing energy in their bodies. These sensations tend to get passed off as something else (ringing in the ear, tingling nerves, increased circulation of blood), but that is only a reflection of how we were taught to perceive our bodies.

In *Spiritual Healing: Energy Medicine for Today* (1991), Jack Angelo writes:

> We have all felt the reassurance, warmth or comfort of another's touch. We have also felt the antagonistic or rejecting touch. There is more, then, to the healing touch than mere gesture. Something is transmitted from one person to another. The healing touch transmits positive energies which can, and do, heal. . . . not only . . . bodies but minds and emotions too.

And in the Fall 1993 issue of *Advances*, the journal of the Fetzer Institute (see Chapter 4), David Aldridge, Ph.D., states:

> [The] notion of "energy field" is the sticking point between orthodox researchers and spiritual practitioners. If such a field exists, researchers maintain, then it should be possible to measure it by physical means, which no one has yet done to the satisfaction of modern science.

The problem probably lies in the use of the word "energy," which has a broader meaning in spiritual healing than it does in physical science, and is likened to organizing principles of vitalism and life force that bring about a harmonizing of the whole person. . . .

What the energy debate misses is the symbolic nature of the healing act, and mirrors the blindness of natural scientific materialism.

Energy Boosting?

Proponents of "alternative" and occult medicine maintain that the "vital force" can be used to prevent, diagnose, and treat disease; improve health and physical fitness; and prolong life. Many also claim that this "energy" and the "physical phase" of the human organism interact through nonphysical entities.

According to yoga philosophy, for example, chakras—transformative vortices or "energy centers"—enable interaction between the body and *prana*, which is the Hindu equivalent of *chi*. Chakras are analogous to the "energy pathways" of acupuncture rather than to acupoints. Although hypothetically there are only five to seven major "body chakras," there is no consensus on the total number; yogis posit hundreds of minor ones. Proponents usually portray chakras as spanning the body from the head to the base of the spine, but there is no consensus on their location or alleged functions. Theosophy, a nonstandard, Eastern-oriented religion pieced together by clairvoyant Helene Petrovna Blavatsky (1831–1891), holds that chakras are the sense organs of the "etheric double." This is supposedly an invisible replica of the physical body that functions as a conductor of "vitality."

Yoga philosophy also posits 107 or 108 *marmas*—points on the skin somewhat similar to acupoints. In *Perfect Health: The Complete Mind/Body Guide* (1990), Deepak Chopra, M.D., (see Chapter 6) advocates a form of massage called marma therapy, which may involve yogic movements and transcendental meditation (TM). He states: "Although they do not usually intersect with prominent blood vessels or nerves, marmas are just as vital, since they mark out where the flow of inner intelligence is moving, indicating spots of maximum sensitivity and awareness."

Occultists maintain that "subtle energy" envelops the human body. This "energy" supposedly constitutes several "subtle bodies"—e.g., a "life-body," a "mortal soul," and an "immortal soul"—or an entity, sometimes layered, whose appellations include: aura (auric field), bioenergy field, bioplasmic body (biofield or bioplasmic force field), doppelganger, etheric body (astral body, dream body, spiritual body, subtle body, or vital body), etheric double, human atmosphere, human energy field, sidereal body (star or astral body), and subtle organizing energy field. For example, anthroposophists—followers of the occult philosophy of Rudolf Steiner (1861–1925)—hold that the human organism consists of a physical body, a vegetal "etheric" body, an animalistic "astral" or "soul" body, and an "ego" or "spirit." Anthroposophical "remedies" purportedly smooth the interaction of these components.

In *Occult Medicine Can Save Your Life* (1985), C. Norman Shealy, M.D., Ph.D., wrote:

> Most [psychics] agree that the aura is three-layered: tight against the skin is a sort of dark layer (some see it as blue or transparent like empty space) a quarter inch or an eighth inch thick; next is a more complicated layer, two to four inches thick and of a blue-gray color which shimmers like heat on a summer highway; and finally there is the fuzzy layer, perhaps light blue, which can be up to several feet thick. Healthy people have bright-colored auras. Disease darkens the aura.

Proponents of aura analysis claim that one's "spiritual skin" is perceptible to clairvoyants and that a special type of photography, termed "Kirlian," can record this "aura." Soviet electrician Semyon D. Kirlian and his wife Valentina developed Kirlian photography—also called corona-discharge photography and "electrography"—in 1939. Kirlian photographers place unexposed film on a metal photographic plate, set an object on the film, and add an electrical field. The resulting photo shows a halo surrounding the outline of the object. Proponents correlate these patterns with acupuncture meridians and claim that "auric" qualities reveal changes in health and emotional state. However, scientific investigators have shown that Kirlian effects depend on the degree of pressure exerted by the subject's body part, the amount of moisture on the body part, the type of photographic paper used, the exposure time, and the photographic development time.

In *Pranic Healing* (1990), chemical engineer Choa Kok Sui, a Filipino of Chinese descent, equates *prana* with *ki*, "vital energy," the "life force," pneuma, mana, and the Hebrew *ruah* (*ruach*)—the "breath of life." He equates pranic healing with psychic healing, magnetic healing, faith healing, "ki healing," "vitalic" healing, and the laying on of hands. Sui states that pranic healing involves the transference of *prana* to heal both the "visible physical body" and the "energy body"—also called the bioplasmic body, etheric body, or etheric double. The "energy body" has an "inner aura," a "health aura," an "outer aura," and organ-like major, minor, and "mini" chakras. Sources of *prana* include sunlight, air, the ground, and trees. "People who are depleted," writes Sui, "tend to unconsciously absorb prana from others. This is why you may have encountered people who tend to make you feel tired or drained for no apparent reason."

According to Sui's method, the "healer" passes at least one hand over the patient's entire body, "scanning" the "inner aura" for "hollows" and "protrusions"—indicating "pranic depletion" and "pranic congestion," respectively. This is followed by "sweeping," wherein the practitioner "cleanses" the patient's aura with both hands. Sweeping allegedly removes "diseased bioplasmic matter," disentangles "health rays," unclogs "meridians," facilitates absorption of *prana*, and "automatically seals holes in the outer aura through which prana leaks out." After sweeping, the "healer" deposits the "diseased bioplasmic matter" removed into a "bioplasmic waste disposal unit"—for example, a bowl of salted water. When it is inconvenient to use such a device, advanced "healers" can visualize a fire and throw the "matter" into it—or simply disintegrate the matter by force of will. Finally, the "healer" simultaneously draws in "air prana" through the chakras and projects *prana* onto the patient's "energy body." A variation of pranic healing involves an invocation to God or to angels. Sui states that proficient healers can effect remote pranic healing. He gives specific instructions for *pranic* treatment of acute appendicitis, acute pancreatitis, cancer, deafness, diabetes, drowning, epilepsy, glaucoma, hepatitis, leukemia, sickle cell anemia, tuberculosis, venereal disease, and other health problems. He also recommends pranic healing to enlarge breasts.

In *Holistic Health Promotion: A Guide for Practice* (1989), Barbara Montgomery Dossey, M.S., writes: "The *universal healing power*, not the healer's personal energy, accomplishes the healing. The *healer* is like a channel . . . permitting the cosmic energy to flow unobstructedly through his or her energy fields into those of the *healee*."

Acu-Nonsense

Acupuncture is a millennia-old practice based on the assumption that *chi* and the physical body interact through a network of many channels or pathways inside the body. Meridians—longitudinal lines on the surface of the body—represent these "pathways." This word "meridians" also refers to the alleged pathways themselves. Acupuncture points—also called acupoints, loci, or *tsubos*—are alleged points of communication between external parts of the body and internal organ-like entities. Acupoints supposedly exist throughout the skin, but some do not lie along the meridians and others lack a specific location. Furthermore, although the classic number of acupoints is 365 (correlated with the number of days in a year), some proponents maintain that the number exceeds two thousand. Acupuncturists insert needles at select points, then rotate the needles or use them to conduct a weak electric current. The mainland Chinese invented "acupuncture anesthesia" (or "acupuncture analgesia") in 1958. Practitioners of another Chinese method, medical Qigong, dispense with needles and allegedly influence their patients' *chi* directly.

In early 1993, a mailing from a Florida company offered a "miraculous" and "revolutionary" product called Acu-Stop 2000—an "acupressure-like device" guaranteed to effect rapid weight loss. The literature tells prospective buyers to wear it on the right ear. It claims that pills, dieting, meal plans, and strenuous exercise are unnecessary. Supposedly, even purchasers with "minimal" willpower need only wear it for a few minutes daily. It allegedly works harmlessly by stimulating—and thus suppressing the activity of—acupoints that regulate appetite. In the same year, self-styled naturopathic physician Richard Minarik of Rego Park, New York, proudly announced his invention of an "incredible" alternative to acupuncture—a plastic clamplike device he calls the "acupresser." A notice claims that one application relieves pain—including arthritis pain, backache, and migraine—for five to six hours and often for three to four days. In August 1993, the price was $45.

Minarik also bills himself as a foot reflexologist. Reflexology is a variant of acupressure. In 1990, he circulated printed material alleging that New York Governor Mario Cuomo had been one of his patients. A photo of Minarik beaming alongside Cuomo near a gas station accompanied the statement: "New York State Governor Mario Cuomo looks very contented after getting his ailing back cured with a foot reflexology treatment from famed foot reflexologist Richard Minarik." However, the governor denied that Minarik had ever treated him. In 1993, Minarik circulated a free booklet that does not refer to Cuomo but counts former President Ronald Reagan, former world heavyweight champion Muhammad Ali, Jackie Onassis, other celebrities, and many Radio City Music Hall dancers as onetime or current patients. The booklet includes a photo of Minarik and Reagan at a microphone and quotes the purportedly grateful president:

> The cramps and spasms in my calf muscles started about two years ago. . . . My personal physician prescribed various medication . . .which wasn't much help. I decided I would try some Foot Reflexology treatments from Foot Reflexologist, Richard Minarik. Mr. Minarik explained to me that crystal-like deposits were building up on the nerve endings in the foot that lead to the calf muscles, and [that] because of this, the calf muscles did not get proper nerve energy and blood circulation which in turn made them contract. Mr. Minarik said he would break up these crystal deposits in my feet and then my calf muscles would function normally.

"Acu-nonsense" appears limitless.

Orgonomy Dreams

Unlike vitalists prone to esotericism, orthodox Reichians take a forthright approach to describing their version of the vital force, called orgone. Wilhelm Reich (1897–1957) was an Austrian-born American psychoanalyst and an associate of Sigmund Freud. He coined the word "orgone" to refer to his hypothetical fundamental, omnipresent, life-sustaining, intelligent radiation. Reich claimed that sexual orgasm released this "primordial cosmic energy" and that orgone supplied power to spaceships (UFOs). He wrote thirty books. In his last, *Contact with Space*, he recounted his alleged efforts to save the earth from alien spacemen. "Orgonomy" refers to Reichian theory and the use of devices that purportedly accumulate and direct orgone. Police officers arrested Reich in 1956 for shipping such devices across state lines. At the age of sixty, he died of a heart attack in a federal penitentiary.

Psychiatrist Elsworth F. Baker, M.D., founded the American College of Orgonomy in 1968. Located in Princeton, New Jersey, the college describes orgonomy as a science that "embraces groundbreaking approaches in psychiatry, medicine, childrearing, social sciences, biology, and atmospheric/environmental research." It promotes "orgone research" and conducts a "postgraduate" training program in medical orgonomy for physicians. Richard Morrock attended the college's 1991 annual meeting and reported the proceedings in the Spring 1992 *Skeptical Inquirer*. One of the speakers described an experiment purportedly showing that temperature changes occurred somewhat more quickly inside a small "orgone accumulator" made of wood and metal than inside a control box made of plastic. Morrock comments: "It was not clear what was proved, other than the already known fact that metal and plastic do not conduct heat at the same rate."

In *The Orgone Accumulator Handbook: Construction Plans, Experimental Use and Protection Against Toxic Energy* (1989), former university professor James DeMeo, Ph.D., describes orgone as "cosmic life energy" that is ubiquitous, mass-free, directly observable and measurable, and "accumulated naturally" by living organisms through eating, drinking, breathing, and the skin. He states that the biological effects of a "strong orgone charge" include tingling and warmth at the surface of the skin, flushing, moderation of blood pressure and pulse rate, and an increase in gastrointestinal activity, tissue growth and repair, immunity, and liveliness. He ascribes to Reich the claim that orgone accumulators could "in a limited way . . . even disintegrate tumors." DeMeo relates how a farmer he met used a "tube accumulator" to cure a "fast-spreading form" of liver cancer expected to kill him in six months. He writes:

It seems that he went back to his doctor, who saw his changed condition and could not find a trace of the liver cancer. The doctor got real mad at him, and accused him of going to some big city hospital for a "wonder drug." He told his doctor about the accumulator, but the doctor didn't believe him. Since this was a small town in the Midwest, the fact that a farmer had survived the death sentence of the town's most reputable doctor, and had even thrived in spite of that death sentence, was the cause of considerable interest and discussion. Presently, I've been told, there's a shortage of steel oil drums, fibreglass, and steel wool in that town, as the man's friends and neighbors are very busy building their own accumulators!

DeMeo's handbook provides step-by-step instructions for building a half-dozen different "orgone accumulating devices," including a blanket, a "garden seed charger," a "shooter wand," and a cubicle for sitting.

A Strange Way to Keep Score

How do vitalistic "healers" judge the results of their ministrations? In *Spiritual Aspects of the Healing Arts* (1985)—a "holistic healing" anthology compiled by Dora Kunz, the clairvoyant co-developer of therapeutic touch—psychiatrist Laurence J. Bendit, M.D., wrote:

> Even so dread a state as the schizophrenic breakdown is now seen as at least potentially therapeutic. As the child with measles develops immunity to that disease, so the schizophrenic may so change inside that he emerges from the ordeal not a wreck but a new man, more integrated to his own deeper nature, more spiritualized.
> And this applies also to death: physical death may result from the release of the healing forces inside a patient. It is not then a tragedy but a triumph for the healing powers.

If acute illness and death are good signs, obviously vitalistic "healers" can't go wrong!

Reading, Writing, and Religion

Scores of schools and other organizations across the United States provide training or indoctrination in vitalistic "healing" methods. For example, the Barbara Brennan School of Healing in East Hampton, New York, offers a four-year "Professional Healing Science Training Program." Apparently, the only prerequisite for admission is attendance at a three-and-a-half-day introductory workshop costing $450. According to an application-flyer, the workshop covers the laying on of hands and the rudiments of perceiving, balancing, and healing the "human energy field." The four-year program covers the "anatomy, physiology and pathology" and the "psychodynamics" of this alleged field and how to: use the "field" to facilitate communication in difficult relationships, develop "high sense perception" to discern illnesses, channel "spiritual guidance" in healing, heal with color and sound, and live within the "Universal Principle of Healing." The school offers continuing education units to nurses and acupuncturists. The flyer, which describes the school as "highly respected," states: "Graduates usually establish their own full practice in Healing Science within six months of graduation, or employ their mastery in their present health care professions."

The Bateman Institute for Health Education in New York City offers classes in "chi-energy" and "natural childbirth," workshops in Qigong, and a certificate program in yoga therapy. According to a flyer, the certificate program welcomes aspiring "therapists" and provides "experience teaching and dealing with difficult and serious rehabilitation cases." The InnerLight Center in Glen Cove, New York, gives instruction in such subjects as *A Course in Miracles*, attunement, past-life regression, polarity balancing, rebirthing, Tibetan pulsing, and therapeutic, "non-trance" channeling.

The East-West College of the Healing Arts in Portland, Oregon, offers massage therapy programs leading to licensure. Courses in massage cover ayurvedic massage, polarity therapy, reiki, shiatsu, therapeutic touch, and *tui na*. The 1992 East-West catalog stated: "One of the marks of a school's excellence is its recognition by accreditation agencies." It boasted full accreditation by six organizations—but none of these is a regional accrediting agency, and the U.S. Department of Education recognizes only one, the Career College Association. The catalog described the Department of Education as a member of the Council on Postsecondary Accreditation (COPA), but did not indicate that COPA does not recognize the Career College Association.

The East West School of Herbalism in Santa Cruz, California, offers a "professional herbalist course" in "herbal medicine"—based partly on the ayurvedic theory of *tridosha* and Chinese yin/yang theory—through correspondence. The question-and-answer section of the school's brochure appears to encourage the unlawful practice of medicine:

> Graduates of this course should be able to incorporate a practice as an herbal consultant. Although the laws relating to health care state that

no unauthorized person may diagnose disease and prescribe medicine, the system of holistic analysis based upon principles of Oriental diagnosis has nothing to do with the Western concepts of pathological disease and so can be used as a basis of practice without infringing on the law.

Further, herbs are given as safe and effective food supplements, not for the treatment of disease, but for restoring and maintaining the harmonious balance of the whole person and thus, maximizing one's innate, natural ability to overthrow disease.

The Oregon School of Herbal Studies in Junction City, Oregon, offers a certification program that includes courses in aromatherapy and flower essence therapy, homeopathy, psychic therapy, and shamanic herbalism.

Some dubious schools do not promote supernaturalism but train students to become "nonprofessional" practitioners. The School of Herbal Medicine of the National Institute of Medical Herbalists in Suquamish, Washington, offers a one-year correspondence course leading to a "Certificate of Proficiency." The school's admission requirements are: "a basic intelligence," the ability to study, and the desire to learn. Academic success supposedly results in the ability to "adequately recognize the everyday ailments of family and friends" and to "give sound advice."

The unaccredited University of Healing in Campo, California—a "metaphysical school" of "spiritual healing"—offers bachelor's, master's, and doctoral "degrees," a "practitioner certificate," and ordination—all by correspondence. The length of the dissertation may be as few as ten pages, but must be "written in the FIRST PERSON, PRESENT TENSE, TOTALLY POSITIVE in its content and format." There are no final exams. According to the syllabus, the school is "accredited by" and "in corporate harmony with" the Church of God Unlimited. It states:

> The first step in proving to ourselves that we really desire to be the master of ourselves is to set aside the necessary tuition donation for the course or even all the courses we wish to take. Once we have *paid* our way at the college, that is behind us and we can concentrate on our lessons. Paying our tuition donation . . . in the very beginning allows our minds to be free to truly apply ourselves on being a master in consciousness. . . .
>
> If the student is sincere, he will have no difficulty to accomplish the [course work].

The American Society of Alternative Therapists (ASAT) in Gloucester, Massachusetts, offers a correspondence course in "holistic health counseling." Graduates receive a "certificate of certification" from ASAT and a diploma in "transformational counseling" from the Institute of Transformational Studies. Lessons cover "biogram therapy," the bubble of light technique, dream therapy, "parts therapy," past-life therapy, psycho-neuro integration (PNI), self-healing, and "practice building." ASAT claims that fifty hours of training is "enough to prepare for a successful career in holistic health counseling." One of its flyers states: "We do not have a grading or pass/fail system. Our procedures are so easy to understand and apply anyone can master them with a little practice."

Pseudocredentialism is rampant. For example, in 1987, Hohm Press of Prescott Valley, Arizona, published the paperback *Food Enzymes: The Missing Link to Radiant Natural Health* by herbalist and "nutritional consultant" Humbart Santillo. The book's text refers to Santillo as "Mr." over a half-dozen times. Yet its cover claims that he holds a "Doctor's degree" from the Concept-Therapy Institute (see Chapter 13), which he purportedly earned after eight years of study, and a "Doctor of Naturopathy" degree. Other "degrees" listed include "Health Practitioner," "Iridology Certificate of Merit," and "Master Herbalist" ("M.H."). In September 1993, I phoned the Concept--Therapy Institute to inquire about Santillo's "Doctor's degree." A representative explained that Santillo had received an "honorary degree for attending all of our courses." She emphasized that this "credential" was "an honorary certificate." She also informed me that the courses Santillo had taken were still available but did not constitute a "doctorate program." She stated that the institute had discontinued the "degree" in the early 1980s to avoid confusing the public.

The following chapter illustrates how born-again "medicine" has gone bigtime in pop culture.

4

Adventures with "Chi": Much Hype, Little Evidence

Throughout the past three years, the American media presented "alternative medicine" as an admirable candidate for mainstream acceptance. One of its most influential forms is traditional Chinese medicine (TCM)—a subject too vast and convoluted to cover thoroughly in this book. Chinese medicine's most conspicuous basic ideas are those of *chi* ("universal life energy," also spelled "qi"), meridians (the alleged channels that contain *chi* in the body), and yin and yang. According to ancient Chinese cosmology, yin and yang are the opposite but complementary cosmic principles or "energy modes" that compose the *tao*—ultimate reality, universal energy, and living in cosmic harmony.

In the Winter 1994 issue of *Skeptical Inquirer*, Asian-studies scholar Peter Huston attributed TCM's survival in China to: (1) the reluctance of the Chinese to abandon part of their national identity, (2) TCM's utility in closing gaps in medical practice, and (3) subjective benefits in a country where psychiatry and general medical practice are underdeveloped.

The preceding chapter deals with *chi*, meridians, acupuncture (which allegedly regulates *chi*), and related theories. This chapter examines two media portrayals of Chinese medicine and describes my visit to a practitioner.

Healing and the Soul

In February 1993, a five-part series on "alternative" medicine titled "Healing and the Mind with Bill Moyers" debuted on public television. Related literature included a "viewer's guide," a "resource guide for the field of mind body health"

37

containing an abridged version of the viewer's guide, and *Healing and the Mind* (1993), a 370-page companion volume published by Doubleday.

In a 1993 *TV Guide* interview, Moyers, a journalist and former White House press secretary, stated:

There's a grass-roots revolution brewing from people who want alternatives to traditional scientific medicine. This is the beginning of a scientific realization that our feelings *do* affect our health. . . . People are beginning to demand help in becoming responsible for their own well-being. Modern medicine has taken that away, by treating us like cars in for tuneups.

The primary source of funding for "Healing and the Mind" was the Fetzer Institute in Kalamazoo, Michigan. The resource guide describes the institute as a nonprofit educational organization promoting research into health-care methods that "utilize the principles of mind-body phenomena." According to the guide, "The institute believes that study of the mind's influence on the body—and the relationship of the body, mind and spirit—can provide the basis for developing scientifically sound approaches for health care that expand the scope of medical science and give individuals greater control over their own health." The institute's 1991 *Report* states that the body "contains a powerful system of energy, which is a key to physical health." Its research activities are purportedly "directed toward exploring the interrelationships between mental, physical, emotional, and spiritual dimensions of health." Other organizations listed in the resource guide include the Academy of Guided Imagery, American Holistic Health Association, American Holistic Medical Association, American Holistic Nurses Association, and World Research Foundation—all of which attempt to steer the public toward nonscientific healthcare and away from science itself.

The guide also recommends books, magazines, and videotapes advocating the Alexander technique, aromatherapy, chiropractic, holotropic breathwork, homeopathy, macrobiotics, the Maharishi Mahesh Yogi's brand of Hindu medicine, music therapy, naturopathy, polarity therapy, *pranayama*, rebirthing, reiki, shamanism, soul retrieval, therapeutic touch, traditional Chinese medicine, transpersonal psychology, and vibrational medicine. The books include *Healing Powers: Alternative Medicine, Spiritual Communities and the State*; *Spiritual Dimensions of Healing, Music and Miracles*; *Nature as Teacher and Healer*; *Where the Mind Meets the Body*; *The Interrelationship Between Mind and Matter*; *Mind Matters: How the Mind and Brain Interact to Create Our Conscious Lives*; *Body, Self and Soul: Sustaining Integration*; and *The Energy Within*. The magazines include *New Age Journal, East West Natural Health,*

The Journal of Transpersonal Psychology, and *Subtle Energies*, which deals with "energies that interact with the human mind and body."

Since 1991, the Fetzer Institute has published *Advances: The Journal of Mind-Body Health*, a quarterly containing dialogues, review articles, research abstracts, book reviews, and other individual commentaries pertaining to "the capacity of mental phenomena to affect physical health." Unlike peer-reviewed scientific journals, *Advances* publishes little or no original research but functions primarily as a forum for proponents.

Chi Whiz

The first episode of "Healing and the Mind," titled "The Mystery of Chi," was filmed in Beijing and Shanghai in the People's Republic of China. Moyers' "guide" was David M. Eisenberg, M.D. Eisenberg, the principal consultant for the series and a Fellow of the Fetzer Institute, is an instructor at Harvard Medical School and a staff internist at Beth Israel Hospital in Boston. In 1979, Eisenberg had begun a yearlong study of traditional Chinese medicine as mainland China's first American medical exchange student since the Cultural Revolution. In 1983, he returned as part of a medical delegation whose primary purpose was to investigate Qigong therapy.

In *Encounters with Qi: Exploring Chinese Medicine*, first published in 1985, Eisenberg narrates his experiences during both periods. The book's foreword was written by Harvard University medical professor Herbert Benson, M.D., who had proposed and attended the 1983 expedition. Benson had also investigated the physiological effects of transcendental meditation in 1968 and had developed his own stress-reduction method, described in his 1975 bestseller *The Relaxation Response*.

In *Encounters with Qi*, Eisenberg relates how his acupuncture instructor, Dr. Zhang, surgically treated a case of severe asthma with neither acupuncture nor an anesthetic: The acupuncturist made a one-inch incision along the breastbone of the nervous young patient and used a clamplike instrument to scrape the exposed surface of the bone. After bandaging the wound, he directed the patient to return in a week for another treatment. Eisenberg told Zhang he thought the procedure was "barbaric." But Zhang claimed that use of an anesthetic would have rendered the treatment ineffective. "If you ask me for proof," he said, "I have only my own experience and the experience of other acupuncturists." Zhang further claimed that the procedure could cure 70 to 80 percent of all asthmatic children. Eisenberg concluded: "There was no way to verify this claim." He adds that the patient did not return for treatment for several weeks. "Zhang," he writes, "assumed this meant her condition had responded to therapy."

"Alternative" Hype

In 1991, the Fetzer Institute supported a study of "unconventional medicine" that was published in January 1993 in *The New England Journal of Medicine* and immediately became a public-relations gold mine for "alternative" health-care. In the study, Eisenberg and several collaborators directed a national telephone survey that asked 1,539 adults about their use of "conventional" and "unconventional" medical services. The article stated that a third of the interviewees had used at least one "unconventional therapy" in 1990. The authors concluded that "unconventional medicine has an enormous presence in the U.S. health care system." However, the study fell far short of demonstrating this claim. First, the researchers counted relaxation techniques, massage, commercial weight-loss programs, self-help group therapy, and biofeedback as forms of "unconventional medicine." None of these approaches is validly inside "unconventional medicine" or outside "conventional" medicine. Second, only 11 percent of the interviewees had reported consulting a provider of "unconventional therapy." All the "unconventional therapy" patients with cancer, diabetes, lung disease, skin problems, high blood pressure, or urinary disease had consulted a medical doctor.

Eisenberg and his colleagues had defined "unconventional therapies" as "medical intervention not taught widely at U.S. medical schools or generally available at U.S. hospitals"—a definition much broader than the usual depiction of "alternative" healthcare. But the press promptly announced that "alternative" medicine was on the rise.

Superforce or Supersuggestibility?

Qigong is an ancient Chinese system involving patterned breathing, posture, stylized movements, visualization, and contemplation. "Qigong" literally means "to work the *Qi* (*chi*)." "*Gong*" is a Mandarin word pertaining to skill. Its Cantonese equivalent is "*kung*," as in "kung fu." In an issue of *Qi: The Journal of Traditional Eastern Health & Fitness*, licensed acupuncturist Nan Lu, founder of the American Taoist Healing Center in New York City and a promoter of Qi gong meridian therapy, states:

> The number of Qigong systems and methods is vast. Chinese masters say that each method provides a different path to the mountain top, or Tao, and that every time Qigong is practiced the path brings the

practitioner a little closer to the peak. However, some paths are quicker than others. While some move rapidly toward the mountain top, others contain detours, or are simply roads that wind around the mountain's base and leave one at the head of a trail that will bring more direct passage.

Lu divides Qigong into three categories: (1) Confucianist Qigong, which centers on behavior and supposedly enhances artistry; (2) Buddhist Qigong, comprising 84,000 systems that center on charitable and pious deeds; and (3) Taoist Qigong, comprising 3,600 systems that center on morality. Lu states that each system of Taoist Qigong has 10,000 techniques.

In *Encounters with Qi*, Eisenberg describes what he calls the major components of Qigong: (1) internal (soft) Qigong as the "manipulation" of *chi* within one's own body through exercise; and (2) external (hard) Qigong as the projection or emission of *chi* from fingertips toward another body, particularly toward acupuncture points. His book includes a photograph provided by a "Qigong master," which depicts the practitioner wearing a surgical mask and gown and aiming two fingers in ray-gun fashion at a patient on an operating table. Eisenberg describes an event wherein another "master"—Dr. Zhou— performed external Qigong on Dr. Benson, who stood amidst an audience in a large room:

> Benson remained motionless, closed his eyes, and performed his own relaxation exercise. Zhou approached him cautiously, then aimed his arm at [Benson's] midsection. Benson appeared very relaxed, almost in a trance. Then he began to move. He swayed a bit from side to side, lost his footing, and tripped. He did not fall, but was clearly off balance. Zhou's arm tracked Benson's every movement. . . . It was impossible to know who was leading whom. Benson then began to twist his hips, first to the right, then to the left. He swiveled 180 degrees with awkward jerks.

Benson moved in a "bizarre" manner for five minutes before Zhou ended the "demonstration." Afterwards, Benson addressed the audience. Eisenberg writes:

> He described the peculiar sensations he had had during the demonstration. One was that of physical pressure seemingly coming from Zhou. In response to this pressure, Benson had voluntarily moved in an effort to resist Zhou's actions and test Zhou's strength. Benson said that he had initiated all of his own movements and was not convinced that Zhou could move him in any direction against his will. . . . In the end the demonstration did little to shake Benson's profound skepticism of man's ability to emit external energy.

In his book, Eisenberg compares Qigong to faith healing, the laying on of hands, and shamanism. He quotes Benson: "It was all too subjective. Judgments cannot be made on the basis of subjective feelings alone. What we need is objective, reproducible data." Eisenberg also described himself as very susceptible to suggestion; Benson, he writes, judged him "extremely hypnotizable."

Perhaps he is gullible as well. People who stand with their eyes closed and feet together usually begin to sway and tend to fall backward. Stage hypnotists often demonstrate this phenomenon and use it (with reinforcing suggestions) to help identify people who are highly suggestible and therefore suitable for hypnosis.

"Shir" Fantasy

In "The Mystery of Chi," Eisenberg makes his entrance in a segment filmed at Dongzhimen Hospital, which he describes as Beijing's largest hospital of traditional Chinese medicine—"probably the most famous in the country." The mainland Chinese, he says, can choose between "two completely separate medical systems": Western medicine and the type practiced at Dongzhimen, which he describes as "purely traditional Chinese medicine with a few pockets of Western medicine here and there." Yet the first person he interviews—a Dongzhimen patient—states she is taking both Western and traditional Chinese medicines. Furthermore, the episode shows another interviewee undergoing surgery for a pituitary tumor—with, according to Eisenberg, a "combination" of "acupuncture anesthesia" and a Western painkiller.

"Healing" does not mention that in American hospitals, surgeons routinely keep patients undergoing such operations awake—without acupuncture—to better monitor developments. In the May 26, 1984 issue of *The Lancet*, Petr Skrabanek, Ph.D., wrote: "The mystery of acupuncture anesthesia largely evaporates when we learn that it was supplemented by a premedication, local anesthesia with procaine, and an intravenous drip with pethidine [a narcotic painkiller] and other drugs, that the patients were carefully selected and perhaps only 10-15% were deemed suitable, and that, despite all this, not all patients obtained adequate analgesia."

What Moyers terms the "strangest" event he witnessed with Eisenberg was a "demonstration" of external Qigong by a teacher called Master Shir. Eisenberg "warns" Moyers: "What Master Shir claims he can do just doesn't look real." Shir alleges he can affect other people's bodies by projecting onto them his "energy"—his thoughts or will. Moyers and

Eisenberg observe him as he apparently: (1) causes one of his students to stumble merely by tapping the younger man's fist once with four of his fingers; (2) zaps the same student with Moyers' hand in-between, making the student jiggle as if his finger were inside an electrical socket; (3) casually dislodges a line of six "assailants"; and (4) resists the attempts of a "hard" martial artist— a robust-looking American man evidently much younger than Shir—to up-heave or throw him. Eisenberg himself remarks: "It doesn't look real." It certainly didn't.

Next, Moyers and Eisenberg watch a doctor performing medical Qigong— sometimes called "acupuncture without needles"—on a patient said to have a brain tumor. Moyers comments that, ostensibly, the Qigong therapist's closest Western relative is the professed "faith healer." Eisenberg asks the doctor how he projects his *chi*. The doctor responds with a proverb: "Some things can be sensed, not explained." He adds: "In order to understand Qigong, you must first cross the threshold. Once inside, you can ask me questions."

This is the standpoint of mysticism, not of science. Yet Eisenberg concludes: "My studies in China have convinced me more and more that to understand health I can't just limit it to studying the physical body, I have to expand it to understanding one's spirit." In early 1993, *USA Today* asked him whether *chi* is a spiritual metaphor or a physical reality. He responded that it was "fun" remaining "undecided, and open to either possibility."

In 1988, five executive members of CSICOP—the Committee for the Scientific Investigation of Claims of the Paranormal—visited Beijing, Shanghai, and Xian for two weeks and tested claims made by Qigong masters and others alleged to have psychic powers. The CSICOP team included professional magician James Randi. After they informed interested Qigong masters that they would conduct the tests under rigorous conditions, several volunteers failed to show up. One whom they did observe—a Dr. Lu—stood about eight feet behind a woman who was lying on a table and moved his arms rhythmically. After the patient began to move, Lu maintained that *qi* was emanating from his fingertips and that the patient's movements were reactions to his efforts. However, when the two were placed in separate rooms, the patient "writhed during the entire session quite independent of what the Qigong master did." The investigators concluded:

> In the context of their roles as master and patient, both knew what was expected of them. They both believed in the power of Qi to make the woman move, hence she moved. It was clear to us that Dr. Lu's movements *followed* those of the patient when they were tested in the same room.

My Own "Encounter" with *Chi*

On September 7, 1993, I went to Son's Acupuncture and Herb Clinic—also called Acupuncture and Tui-Na Clinic—in Woodside, New York. Signs on the outside of the two-story building invite passersby to experience "Chinese Medicine, a natural approach to health care." The clinic's operator, Hye Min Son, "O.M.D."—"Doctor of Oriental Medicine"—provided me with a free consultation. In broken English, Son stated that he had obtained his "O.M.D." degree upon completion of an unaccredited program in California, but that he also held a master's degree in acupuncture from an accredited school in the same state. He added that he had studied law in Korea for five years before settling in the United States. "I don't like lawyers," he said.

The consultation lasted about an hour. Son did not ask me to fill out a patient questionnaire until nearly forty-five minutes had passed, during which he had made several unpleasant allegations about my health. He began the consultation by asking: "What's your problem?" I informed him that I had moderate periodontal (gum) disease, virtually without symptoms. I explained that I had had the condition for about fifteen years but that it had worsened recently. I added that I was a writer with a degree in health science developing a book on "alternative" medicine. Later, in response to different questions, I specified my only other active "health problems": thinning of the hair on my head, mild indigestion following consumption of dairy products, occasional dizziness upon standing (postural hypotension), and coldness in my hands and feet during winter.

Son declared that "thinking too much . . . a lot of stress" was one of my problems. He said I had a severe deficiency of *chi* in my spleen and that it affected my stomach since the spleen (yin) and stomach (yang) are complementary organs. He further pronounced my internal organs prematurely old. Although I had not said I was tired—and, in fact, was not—Son told me I was "feeling tired" in my muscles and bones because my spleen and stomach were not spreading "nutrition." He construed the tendency of my hands and feet to become cold as "low, low blood," asserting that my spleen was not producing enough blood.

In traditional Chinese medicine, "pulse diagnosis" is the examination of the pulse to discover the condition of internal organs. Like scientific physicians, practitioners of Chinese medicine use the radial artery at the wrist. However, whereas scientific practitioners take one pulse at either wrist to determine rate and rhythm, "traditionalists" seek six pulses at each wrist. These pulses allegedly correspond to twelve internal spheres of bodily function. To describe the pulses, practitioners of Chinese medicine use such terms as: bolstering-like, confined, empty, floating, flooding, full, knotted, leather, sinking, slippery, soggy, tight, and wiry. A "wiry" pulse, for example, supposedly indicates liver disease.

After checking my pulse at both wrists, Son stated that my capacity to hold *chi* was low and that I had "a lot of problems." He said my pulse was rapid because of a deficiency of yin or an excess of yang. He claimed that "yin is material" and that blood and water contain it. He said that yang was invisible, like air or power.

Son stated that his aim was to "tonify" my spleen and stomach, not with acupuncture but with herbs—whose effects he claimed were longer. He also asserted that the herbs were "powerful" and would increase yin without side effects. He stated that I had to take them for "a long time" and that the performance of my spleen, stomach, and kidneys would not improve quickly. But he added that I would probably feel much better within two months.

Son removed a small, sealed bottle from a cabinet. It was labeled "Ginseng and Astragalus Combination." He transferred the entire contents— a week's supply of 128 tablets—to a small plastic bag that bore a pharmacy logo and stated (in Mandarin): "Secure [or safe] • reliable • no side effects." The cost was $45. Son instructed me to take eighteen of the pills daily, six at a time. He claimed that they were unavailable in stores, even in Chinatown, and that they were a "prescription" product. I followed his directions. The pills were neither tasty nor easy to swallow. If they had any palpable effect, it was tiredness.

My "Encounter" with Qigong

On the evening of October 20, 1993, I attended a free Qigong workshop at the American Taoist (or Daoist) Healing Center in New York City's Chinatown with a friend who was born and raised in mainland China. The center offers acupressure, "Daoist energy reflexology," herbal therapy, and a three-year curriculum that includes courses in tai chi, Qigong, and the use of spears and swords. A flyer designed for mailing states that only a qualified teacher can open acupuncture channels and increase and improve a student's "life force."

Besides staffers and students, about thirty people attended the workshop, which consisted of an introduction by orthopedic surgeon Robert Feldman, M.D., four testimonial speeches, a Qigong demonstration, a talk by founder/ director Nan Lu, O.M.D., group practice of Qigong, and a question-and-answer session. Feldman translated "Qigong" as "energy work" and asserted that *chi* is discoverable in both animate and inanimate matter. Yet he stated: "I've practiced it for fifteen years and only . . . on two occasions did I feel something happen that I was sure was not myself consciously doing it. . . . something moving inside of me that was beyond or out[side] of my own volition."

The first testimonial speaker said that, as a longtime meditator, she had turned to Qigong after a quick sequence of personal tragedies. The second speaker, named Irma, stated that she had turned to Qigong after suffering a nervous breakdown. She said she had needed two things before "finding" Qigong: "more energy . . . to think properly" and "magic"—"something from the outside, something given to me . . . that I felt that I did not have myself." Irma stated: "The first time that I saw a [Qigong] demonstration . . . I just felt I had the answer." The third testimonial speaker gushed:

I worked at a place that had air conditioning in the summer, and it was so cold that . . . I would get chilled to the bone. I think the second summer, after taking Qigong . . . for about a year and a half, I noticed . . . that . . . my hands might get cold and my nose would get cold, but the body wouldn't get cold. It was the most remarkable thing for me. . . . I thought, whatever is happening is just remarkable, that I feel the warmth in my body.

At the outset of his talk, Nan Lu cited what he called a Taoist principle: "Just do whatever you need to do." He described the human body as a small universe and declared: "Once you connect with the universe, you can live forever." He further stated:

You have to find a way you can connect together. . . . We think the body has two kinds of bodies: one is the energy body; one is the physical body. So physical body is the house or place that the energy body will stay. So if [it is a] big house or you don't take care your house . . . your energy body will slip away. . . . Energy body [will go to] the other place. So that's why . . . a lot of people heard about the past life. What does "past life" mean? It means your energy body already [went to another] place. . . .

Qigong . . . makes your energy body and your physical body connect together. But most times our energy body and the physical body are not together. So that's why we have a lot of problems— physical problems and personal problems. . . . And sometimes when we have problems, we cannot pick ourselves up. . . . We don't have enough energy to support the physical body. . . . We don't have enough power to support the physical body. . . .

Energy body is invisible. . . . So people all in America . . . everybody want proof. . . . They want to see the proof about . . . *chi* . . . because until now, [after] almost four thousand years . . . still nobody can prove what is really *chi*. . . . Real things never can be proved. . . . The energy is more faster than the science. . . .

If the [particular Qigong] system can pass... three thousand years, it's got to be good.

In response to a question, Lu said that Qigong and yoga were very similar, but he added that "good Qigong is more [beneficial] than bad yoga." In response to another question, he stated that Qigong practitioners eventually become vegetarians.

The first group Qigong exercise involved slow movements and was a pleasant way of stretching. However, the second exercise consisted of standing still for about seven minutes with legs slightly bent and forearms held horizontal. For most of this time, someone played a piano.

Toward the end of the workshop, an attendee asked Lu if he knew Qigong practitioners who had achieved exceptional longevity. Lu replied that he knew someone who had reached the age of two hundred. The same inquirer asked where the alleged person lived. "He lives in the mountain," answered Lu. My companion said he found Lu amusing. I agree. The personableness of gurus is at least as important as the mystique of the products they sell.

A Lot of Balls

Does it take balls to improve one's health? Some proponents of traditional Chinese medicine seem to think so. Acu-ball pressure is a form of self-applied acupressure characterized by the use of soft, solid-rubber balls. Much more popular is the practice of manually rotating "Chinese health balls," also called "Qi Gong balls," Chinese reflex balls, and reflex balls. These come in four sizes (one for children) and various forms, including hollow enamel balls, hollow metal balls with a ball inside, solid jade balls, solid marble balls, and magnetic balls. Variants include "bubble balls," which are elastic and have conical protuberances; "twin balls," which resemble a dumbbell; and "musical balls," such as the brass "yin-yang ball." In *Chinese Health Balls: Practical Exercises* (1990), Hans Höting writes that musical balls are rotated in the hand or worn on a chain around the neck. He claims that their "therapeutic value" lies in the "mantra sound" they make when they move. Höting's 107-page book features a "Health Diary"—nineteen blank pages he calls "Your Own Memorandum of Fun and Progress." Pacific Spirit Corporation, a mail-order house in Forest Grove, Oregon, sells the book and the balls. A 1993 catalog claims:

> Playing with a pair of Reflex Balls will not only keep your hands & fingers limber but will help balance Right & Left Brain consciousness.
> ... Reflex Balls have been used in China for centuries. In Chinese

medicine they are believed to benefit the brain and nervous system, improve memory, stimulate blood circulation, relax the muscles and joints, tone the internal organs and balance the chi (life energy). They are also used for prevention and treatment of arthritis and hypertension. In each chrome plated ball is a chime which adds a beautiful effect when the balls are rotated.

The Bottom Line

Advocates of "alternative" medicine say that client satisfaction—which can be considerable—proves that their theories are correct. Some also claim that their methods are useful adjuncts to scientific medical care. But William T. Jarvis, Ph.D., professor of preventive medicine at Loma Linda University in California and president of the National Council Against Health Fraud, sees it differently. In response to the "Healing and the Mind" television series, he stated:

> What they don't say is that the "true believers" and the charlatans don't really help the desperate beyond giving them attention. Massage feels great, but what does it do inside? Herbal remedies can have natural stimulants and tranquilizers, but people think something special is going on inside their bodies. The old snake-oil salesmen used to lace their potion with opium or alcohol, and people liked that, too.

I certainly agree. Besides being inconsistent with one another, supernaturalistic "healing" practices do not complement, elucidate, or run parallel to scientific healthcare. Rather, they obscure and conflict with sound treatment.

Part II

"Spiritual Healing"

5

Hindu "Healing":
Yoga and Ayurveda

Yoga and ayurveda are the broad, overlapping "healing" systems that have developed within the ancient religious tradition of Hinduism and spawned many "up-to-date" mystical methods and products. Proponents acclaim them as having passed the "test of time" with flying colors. They are the superstars of "spiritual healing."

What is Spiritual Healing?

I use the term "spiritual healing" to encompass health-centered systems and methods that affirm the idea of "life after death" and borrow conspicuously from religious traditions. However, the term has divergent meanings. For example, it may refer to faith healing. The *1992–1993 Holistic Health Directory*, published by *New Age Journal*, states:

> Practitioners of spiritual healing work on the patient's "spiritual body," sometimes with the assistance of "helpers"—including power animals, angels, inner teachers, the patient's higher self, or other spiritual forces. The practitioner—be it priest, shaman, or soul retriever—does not generally claim to be directly responsible for the healing. Instead, the practitioner views his or her role as a conductor of healing energy or forces from the spiritual realm.

The term "spiritual healing" can also refer to spirit healing, a form of channeling whose advocates claim that healing is the work of divine power or deceased doctors who have not let death stand in the way of their practice. Of course, it is convenient for "spiritual healers" and mediums to insist that they are not the source of healing but merely a pipeline for the Holy Spirit or some other discarnate entity—for if this were so, there would be nobody to blame for treatment failures except the patient, whom the practitioner may accuse of having insufficient faith.

"Spiritual healing" is based on four assumptions: (1) the ultimate source of healing is supernatural; (2) this source is usable directly by the ill person, through other persons, and/or through intermediary supernatural entities; (3) death indicates the beginning of a transition either to an afterworld or to another incarnation; and (4) all human beings are paranormally or supernaturally interconnected. This book focuses on yoga, ayurveda, macrobiotics, and the Edgar Cayce tradition, but there are many other spiritual approaches, including anthroposophical medicine, Christian evangelical healing, Christian Science, exorcism, shamanism, Sufi healing, and Tibetan medicine.

One of spiritual healing's major lures is the mystic "conversion" or "awakening." In *Direct Healing*, first published in 1916, Paul Ellsworth foreshadowed the expressions of present-day spiritual healing:

> There is a spirit in man, latent usually, but which may be quickened and made positive and dominant in the life. When this quickening takes place, the individual ceases to be an insulated unit, at variance with every other unit, and becomes one with that Universal Spirit which permeates and controls all things. Such a man becomes truly a wonder-worker, for he is filled with wisdom and power, and with that broad and tolerant sympathy which brings him into harmony with the soul of things.

As a teenager, and even as a young adult, I fantasized that a momentous change—requiring of me little or no effort—would overtake my personality. Today I understand that this was the escapist thinking of a directionless malcontent.

The Striving for Nothingness

Hinduism is a complex of sociocultural and religious beliefs and practices that evolved on the Indian subcontinent. Hinduism is over three thousand years old. Its main features are: (1) yoga; (2) a system of hereditary classes (castes); (3) the view that all forms ("essential natures") and theories are aspects of a unique external being (supernaturalistic pantheism); and (4) beliefs in nonviolence (ahimsa), karma, the obligation of the individual to fulfill caste function and divine law (dharma), reincarnation (passing of the alleged soul into a new human body or another life-form), and nirvana.

"Karma" literally means "deed." In Hinduism, Buddhism, and other oriental religions, karma is the total effect of one's actions over all of one's incarnations. The supreme goal of Hinduism is nirvana—the highest form of *samadhi* (mystical ecstasy or "superconsciousness"). "Nirvana" literally means "extinction." In Hinduism, the term refers to complete detachment from the material world, which entails termination of the "essentially unpleasant and painful" cycle of birth, life, death, and rebirth. It also refers to union with the impersonal "world spirit," a condition devoid of personality.

The goal of Zen Buddhism is satori (or *kensho*)—a state of "enlightenment" or "spiritual awakening" somewhat comparable to *samadhi*. Satori is characterized by irrationality, impassivity, and the equivalent of a superiority complex. The alleged end product of the deepening of *satori* is the condition called "no-mind." *The Shambhala Dictionary of Buddhism and Zen* explains: "In the experience of enlightenment there is no distinction between knower and known." In *Zen Macrobiotics*, George Ohsawa defined satori as "the tangible and logical conviction that [one] has arrived, body and soul, in the kingdom of freedom, happiness and justice." However, the *Zen Dictionary* (1972) states: "If the experience can be characterized either mentally or emotionally it is not *the* satori."

The Cornucopia of Yoga

"Yoga" derives from a Sanskrit word (*yogah*) that literally means "yoke" and implies a harnessing of oneself to God. Yoga is the Hindu means of achieving nirvana. It features a method of inward concentration consisting of psychosomatic practices. These include postures (*asanas*), breathing exercises (*pranayama*), and a mental exercise (*pratyahara*) designed to facilitate withdrawal from unpleasant stimuli.

Like acupuncture and Qigong, yoga has many variants. *Pranayama* and kundalini are among their most important themes. "*Pranayama*" refers to breathing exercises yogis perform to control *prana*—the "life force"—and to produce an altered state of consciousness. "Kundalini" literally means "coiled." Believers liken kundalini to a snake coiled at the base of the spine and often refer to it as the "serpent power." They hold that kundalini is primordial cosmic energy and that it is ordinarily dormant. However, yogic practices such as *pranayama* allegedly can activate it. Depending upon the individual's skill and wisdom, activation of kundalini supposedly results in enlightenment, madness, malignant disease, enfeeblement, or death.

The major schools or aspects of yoga and their foci are: (1) *hatha* yoga—controlling the physical body through postures, *pranayama*, and "purification" practices (*kriyas*); (2) *laya* yoga—kundalini, the chakras, and bodily sounds audible when the ears are covered; (3) mantra (or *nada*) yoga—mind control; (4) *jnana* (or *nana*) yoga—understanding the laws of the universe; (5) bhakti yoga—devotion to a god; (6) karma yoga—selfless service, duty, and behavior control; and (7) *raja* (*ashtanga* or *astanga*) yoga, which encompasses all the foregoing schools.

Other forms of yoga include *adhayatma* (or *adhyata*) yoga, Bikrams yoga, dharma yoga, *dhyana* yoga, dream yoga, *ghatastha* yoga, *ishta* yoga, Iyengar yoga, *japa* yoga, *jivamukti* (or *jivanmukti*) yoga, *kripalu* yoga, lama yoga, *l'chaim* yoga, polarity yoga, *samadhi* yoga, *yantra* yoga, integral yoga™ (*purna* yoga), *kriya* yoga, agni yoga, tantric yoga (Shakti yoga), and kundalini yoga. "*Adhayatma*" means "supreme self." Practitioners of *adhayatma* yoga supposedly "overcome" identification with their bodies and minds. Dharma yoga centers on religious duties. *Dhyana* yoga is a mental discipline that often involves attainment of a trance. Dream yoga is a set of Tibetan methods for producing "lucidity" in dreaming (awareness that one is dreaming). "*Ishta*" literally means "beloved," "desire," or "chosen." Alan Finger, who established yoga schools in Los Angeles and New York City, founded *ishta* yoga. B.K.S. Iyengar developed Iyengar yoga, a system involving postures and *pranayama*. "*Japa*" refers to the process of repeating a sacred name or formula—vocally, mentally, or by moving one's lips silently. *Kripalu* yoga is a variant of hatha yoga that emphasizes meditation. Lama yoga is one of the methods of Astara, a "reborn mystery school" and nondenominational Christian church in Upland, California. Lama yoga supposedly safely "awakens" kundalini. *L'Chaim* yoga is a Judaic variant of *kripalu* yoga, involving chakra healing, Jewish melodies, and *makko-ho*—a mode of stretching based on traditional Chinese medicine. Polarity yoga is a mode of polarity balancing (see Chapter 10). *Samadhi* yoga is a mode of bodywork that puirportedly tranquilizes the subconscious and causes "core tissues" to "bloom." Yantra yoga, a Tibetan Buddhist variant of hatha yoga, emphasizes continuous movement.

"Integral yoga" is the trademark for a system founded by Sri Ghose Aurobindo (1872–1950) and promoted by Sri Swami Satchidananda. The swami's organization, Integral Yoga International, established in 1966, describes integral yoga as a synthesis of hatha yoga, karma yoga, raja yoga, bhakti yoga, *jnana* yoga, and japa yoga. The goal of integral yoga is twofold: the ascent of the "human spirit" to the divine and the integration of the divine with the workaday world.

From Sacrificial Fire to Flames of Passion

Kriya yoga is the spiritual path fostered by Paramahansa Yogananda (1893-1952), who founded the Self-Realization Fellowship in Los Angeles in 1925. *"Kriya"* literally means "deed," "operation," or "effort." In his bestselling "spiritual classic," *Autobiography of a Yogi*, first published in 1946, Yogananda described kriya yoga as the eternal science of "God-realization"—a "fire rite" whereby yogis can spare *prana* and thus arrest bodily decay. Yogananda apparently took to heart the maxim "Cleanliness is next to godliness." He wrote:

> The yogi casts his human longings into a monotheistic bonfire consecrated to the unparalleled God. This is indeed the true yogic fire ceremony, in which all past and present desires are fuel consumed by love divine. The Ultimate Flame receives the sacrifice of all human madness, and man is pure of dross. His metaphorical bones stripped of all desirous flesh, his karmic skeleton bleached by the antiseptic sun of wisdom, inoffensive before man and Maker, he is clean at last.

Yogananda described his theory of healing in *Scientific Healing Affirmations*: (1) disease stems from the inaction of the "life force" or "life energy" within the ill; (2) sick persons prolong their illness through habitual negative thinking; and (3) words spoken repeatedly with "sincerity, conviction, faith, and intuition" by the ill can "move the Omnipresent Cosmic Vibratory Force to render aid."

Agni yoga—also called actualism and fire yoga—is a spinoff developed in the 1950s by American-born Russell Paul Schofield, a theistic clairvoyant with doctorates in psychology, naturopathy, and divinity. "Agni" is the name of the eternally young Hindu god of fire, the banisher of evil spirits. The word also refers to the ayurvedic "fire element"—one of the five *mahabhutas*, whose symbols are earth, water, fire, air, and space. Actualism involves the laying on of "lighted" hands and supposedly burns off "psychic residues." The New York Actualism Center, on the upper West Side, describes actualism as "training in the use of energy tools and techniques of 'inner light fire,' in which light illuminates the darkened areas of consciousness, and consuming fires eliminate the conditions that obstruct awareness and separate us from ourselves and others." In *Maps of Consciousness* (1971), Ralph Metzner listed actualism's "laws of energy": (1) thought directs energy; (2) energy follows thought; (3) mild obstructions to energy flow cause discomfort and strong obstructions cause pain and "dis-ease"; and (4) energy concentrates where one focuses thought. Besides the Manhattan center, there are five actualism centers, all in California.

Tantric yoga—also called tantra or tantrism—developed in the third and fourth centuries C.E. While the major schools of yoga hold that carnal desires impede the pursuit of nirvana, tantra holds that they are potential vehicles. Tantrics seek to arouse the goddess Shakti—"divine feminine energy" symbolized by the kundalini serpent—through ritualized sexual intercourse. The Hawaiian Goddess Source School of Tantra Yoga, on Maui, offers seminars, audiotapes, and videotapes on tantra. A flyer from the school states: "Tantra uses techniques of sexual healing, breath control, transformative touch, varied positions, energy exchange meditations and unique advanced lovemaking techniques." Kundalini yoga shares with tantric yoga the goal of "kundalini awakening."

Keith Kornhorst attended a weekend workshop on "tantric sex" with his girlfriend and reported his experience in the March/April 1993 issue of *Natural Health*. Margo Anand, author of *The Art of Sexual Ecstasy: The Path of Sacred Sexuality for Western Lovers* (1989), conducted the workshop. Kornhorst writes:

> Anand admits that her brand of Westernized Tantra would amuse the Tibetan monk. "He'd probably laugh in my face and tell me I don't know the first thing about it," she said. "Tantra means years and years of purifying one's emotions and spiritual being before even touching the sexual aspect of Tantra. But I like taking shortcuts." . . .
>
> In Tantra, men are taught to forestall ejaculation. Anand did not specifically instruct the men how to do this, but the idea is that just prior to orgasm, men are to take that energy and "direct" it through the body instead of letting it out through ejaculation. . . .
>
> I don't think what we did was truly Tantra. . . . The retreat lacked a spiritual foundation.

Ayurveda

Ayurveda encompasses aromatherapy, astrology, diet, herbalism, massage, and numerous other methods. In approximately the first century C.E., a physician named Charaka (also spelled "Charak" and "Caraka") wrote the first of the two classic ayurvedic texts. About a century later, the surgeon Sushruta (also spelled "Susruta") composed the second text. Both authors claimed that ayurveda is divine in origin. Time-Life Books' *Powers of Healing* relates the following anecdote.

A student once asked Charaka if it were true that "diet is half of

Ayurveda." "No, that is wrong," the great physician is supposed to have said, "it is almost all of Ayurveda."

"Ayur" derives from the Sanskrit *"ayus,"* meaning "life" or "life span." *"Ayu"* means "life" or "daily living." Interpretations of the word *"veda"* include "knowledge," "knowing," "science," "sacred teaching," and "sacred lore." In *Ayurveda: The Science of Self-Healing* (1985), ayurvedic practitioner Dr. Vasant Lad states:

> The science of Ayurveda is based not on constantly changing research data, but on the eternal wisdom of the *rishis* [clairvoyant sages] who received this science, expressive of the perfect wholeness of Cosmic Consciousness, through religious introspection and meditation. Ayurveda is a timeless science. . . .
>
> Ayurveda is truly a holistic science, one in which the sum of many elements comprises its Truth. To question details before a strong overview of the whole science is acquired will prove unproductive and unsatisfactory.

Ayurveda is rooted in the fundamental scriptures of Hinduism—four Sanskrit books called the *Vedas*: the *Rig-veda*, the *Sama-veda*, the *Yajur-veda*, and the *Atharva-veda*. The Aryans—invaders of India in the second millennium B.C.E.—settled in Punjab and compiled the *Vedas* before 500 B.C.E. Orthodox Hindus maintain that these books are eternal and that seers originally beheld their "text" by intuition.

The oldest and most venerated *Veda* is the *Rig-veda*. "Prophets" composed this collection of 1,028 hymns between 1500 and 900 B.C.E. They addressed most of the hymns to various gods—especially the war-god Indra and the fire-god Agni—but directed one to frogs. During complex official rites, priests and sages sang these hymns, prepared a hallucinogenic drink (the juice of a plant called *soma*), ingested it, and made burnt offerings of animals. The *Rig-veda* includes an invocation against rivals: "Whoever has spoken against me with false words when I was acting with a pure heart, O Indra, let him become nothing even as he talks about nothing, like water grasped in one's fist."

The *Sama-veda* and the *Yajur-veda* are how-to books for priests specializing in sacrificial rites. *Free Inquiry* has reported that in 1993, about eight thousand Hindus participated in such a ritual, topped it off with chants designed to prevent natural calamities, and ate the decomposed meat of the animals. At least sixteen devotees died and 630 became ill.

The last of the *Vedas*, the *Atharva-veda*, features magical formulas, curses, and mystical hymns. The composers addressed some of the hymns to deifications of desire, time, and *prana*, the "breath of life." More than a hundred hymns relate to putative botanical cures for various maladies—including conditions supposedly due to demons, ghosts, and gods. "Remedies" and "preventives" include amulets, exorcism, invocations, and other incantations. Vedic medicine developed as a combination of magico-religious and empirical views and practices. The purported causes of disease include sin, violation of a norm, the unjust cursing of a fellow man, and the wrongs committed by one's parents or by "oneself" in a previous incarnation. Disease is either punishment meted out by the gods—directly or through demons—or the result of witchcraft.

In the early nineteenth century, T.A. Wise, a European physician whose avocation was medical history, translated parts of several Sanskrit medical manuscripts in Bengal, India. In *The Hindu System of Medicine*, he described the ayurvedic belief that both good and bad spirits cause disease. Which devil is to blame depends on the physical, emotional, and behavioral characteristics of "possessed" patients and their preferences regarding food, clothing, and place of residence.

Ayurveda has eight or nine major branches: (1) internal (general) medicine; (2) surgery; (3) treatment of diseases of the head and neck—ophthalmology and otolaryngology; (4) toxicology—the treatment of poisoning; (5) psychotherapy or psychiatry—e.g., treatment of seizures supposedly caused by evil spirits; (6) pediatrics; (7) geriatrics, including rejuvenation therapy; (8) aphrodisiac or "virilization" therapy; and, according to some scholars, (9) *panchakarma* ("purificatory procedures"). Today, only internal medicine, geriatrics, aphrodisiac therapy, and *panchakarma* are used extensively.

"*Pancha*" means "five," and "*karma*" means "actions" or "processes." *Panchakarma* consists of emesis therapy ("therapeutic vomiting"), purgation therapy (evacuation of the bowels with a laxative), decoction (watery) enema therapy, oily enema therapy, and nasal insufflation therapy (also called errhine therapy, nasal medication, and nasal administration). Nasal insufflation therapy is the use of medicines that promote or induce nasal discharge. Other ayurvedic treatments include fat therapy (also called oleation therapy and unctuous therapy), sweating therapy (also called sweat therapy and sudation therapy), and bloodletting. Fat therapy involves external application and/or ingestion of fatty substances such as vegetable oils, cod liver oil, milk, ghee (a solid or semifluid clarified butter), and bone marrow.

Ayurvedic "diagnosis" involves examination of the eyes, face, lips, tongue, and nails. Ayurvedists associate parts of the lips and tongue, for example, with internal organs and hold that discolorations, lines, cracks, and irritability in various areas indicate disorders in "corresponding" organs.

Ghostly Forces

The principal ayurvedic theory—called *tridosha*—holds that five "elements" (*mahabhutas*) constitute the human body: earth, air, fire, water, and ether (space). The preponderance of these elements determines various constitutional types, each prone to ailments due to a deficiency or excess of one or more elements. The fundamental constitutional types are *pitta, kapha,* and *vata.* These terms also designate the fundamental physiological forces—humors (body fluids) or *doshas (dosas)*—postulated to characterize the types. *Pitta*— "fire" or "bile"—supposedly combines fire and water. *Kapha*—"mucus," "phlegm," or "water humor"—supposedly combines earth and water. *Pitta* and *kapha* are analogous to the yang and yin of Chinese cosmology (see Chapter 7). *Vata* (or *vayu*)—"wind" or "air humor"—supposedly combines air and "space" and mediates between *pitta* and *kapha.* Ayurvedists identified the *doshas* with the three supposed universal forces: sun, moon, and wind. Tibetan medicine shares several theories with ayurveda, including *tridosha* theory, and involves gods, evil spirits, and fate.

Fundamentals of Ayurvedic Medicine (1989) associates "aggravation" of each *dosha* with the following symptoms.

Vata: coldness, colic, contraction, dryness, fractures, malaise, numbness, punching pain, roughness, skin discoloration, abnormal movements of the limbs, and emaciation (extreme thinness, especially as a result of starvation)

Pitta: anger, burning sensation, discharge of pus, fainting, fatigue, foul smell, giddiness, incoherent speech, stickiness, sweating, and yellowing of the body

Kapha: coldness, "excessive exudation," heaviness, itching, paleness, swelling, unctuousness, inserting physiological waste products into bodily openings, feeling as if one is covered with a wet cloth, and feeling as if "some extraneous material" is adhering to the body

This text, published in New Delhi, was written by Vaidya Bhagwan Dash, Ph.D., a former deputy advisor to India's Ministry of Health and Family Welfare. According to Dash, bloodletting, ghee, milk, moonlight, purgatives, and embracing "females" alleviate aggravation of *pitta*; emetics, errhines, exercise, fighting, sexual indulgence, smoking, "spitting therapy," and sun exposure alleviate aggravation of *kapha*; and bathing, enemas, massage, rest, and sun exposure alleviate aggravation of *vata.*

Robert E. Svoboda, an American who lives in India, received his "medical" degree from an ayurvedic college in India. He offers a correspondence course in ayurveda through The Ayurvedic Institute in Albuquerque, New Mexico. In *Ayurveda: Life, Health and Longevity* (1992), Svoboda states: "The Three Doshas are 'ghosts' (spirits that possess) created by Nature in order to permit embodied life to exist. They do not really belong on the physical plane any more than ghosts do, and yet they remain here working for us; it is no surprise that they can quickly become disturbed." He further writes:

> When either disease or cause is unsure, treatment can still proceed according to the general treatment for the *dosha* involved, since the *doshas* are the prime causes of physical health and disease. Even in diseases of non-physical origin, such as those fevers that are caused by the planets, curses or black magic, the *doshas* must still be identified and rebalanced.

Svoboda describes ayurvedic treatment:

> Disease therapy is a sort of spiritual advancement. Your visit to your healer is a pilgrimage, at the culmination of which comes the healing ritual performed by the doctor-guru, which helps remove your "sins," dietary and otherwise, from where you have stored them, deep within you in the form of *ama*, so that the body's fire element can cleanse you of them. Every moment your body creates your past as it absorbs the products of digestion. By dealing with your past in your present, you can proceed confidently towards your future, a future of righteousness, in which your tissues will be pure and healthy, your wastes quickly and efficiently excreted, and your *doshas* balanced.

Cure for an "Intellectual Headache"?

Ayurveda unifies magical forms of nutrition and pharmacology. In *Ayurveda: The Indian Art of Natural Medicine and Life Extension* (1990), Viennese pharmacist Birgit Heyn states: "As far as Ayurveda is concerned . . . any disharmony in the body can be treated by what we eat. Foods are remedies, plants are healing drugs, and diet is the best therapy."

Ayurveda holds that *prana*—the "life force"—is absorbable from food and the atmosphere. Svoboda writes: "Ideally your food should be grown in your own field or garden so that you have full control over what physical and mental inputs it imbibes. . . . All food should be 'alive' so that it can give life to its eater." The main ayurvedic foods are grains, ghee, and certain vegetables. Svoboda describes eating as "Ayurveda's fire sacrifice, a daily offering of food into the sacred fire of digestion for the purpose of maintaining microcosmic harmony." A 1993 issue of *To Your Health*, published by the Maharishi Ayur-Ved Foundation, lists eight guidelines for improving digestion, according to which: ice-cold foods and drinks dampen the "digestive fire" (*agni*), and warm milk, ghee, ripe fruits, fruit juices, rice, almonds, and dates are "especially nourishing for everyone." Its cover report states:

> When your agni is potent, your body processes food efficiently, distributes all the necessary nutrients to every cell, and burns off and eliminates waste products without leaving any toxins behind. If your agni is feeble, however, it doesn't completely metabolize your food. It creates a sticky, white, toxic substance called *ama*. Ama is undigestible and blocks the channels in the body, inhibiting the normal functioning of Vata, Pitta and Kapha. . . . And because ama contributes to the early stages of many diseases—from arthritis to the common cold—it is essential to keep your agni strong and your digestion healthy.

Ayurvedic nutrition centers on "constitutional type" (*prakruti*), specific food characteristics, and the season of the year. The most important guide to the therapeutic effect of a food purportedly is its "taste": bitter, pungent, astringent, salty (saline), sour, or sweet. In *Diet and Nutrition: A Holistic Approach* (1982), Rudolph Ballentine, M.D., states: "The Ayurvedic pharmacology of taste is essentially a way of putting into formal terms the intuitive and experiential sense of what is right and proper to eat at any moment." In a videotape titled "Fundamentals of Maharishi Ayur-Veda: Natural Healthcare for the Rejuvenation of Mind and Body," Stewart Rothenberg, M.D., stated:

> In general, our desires [for particular foods] can be trusted. And what we find is that over time, as we continue to follow Ayur-Vedic recommendations, we get more and more in tune with our body's needs and [develop] almost a sixth sense with respect to the taste of the food . . . the smell of the food, the quality of the food. We can in fact begin to rely more and more on our own inner sense of what is good for us, because we will be more in touch with balance within and how it relates to the food that we are eating.

A food's "taste" supposedly indicates whether it will increase or decrease a particular *dosha*. However, ayurvedic nutrition involves other food characteristics, which pertain to such factors as adhesiveness, temperature, texture, weight, and "emmoliency" (oily versus moist and dry). For example, cold foods purportedly decrease *pitta*, and oily foods supposedly increase *kapha*. *Ayurveda: The Science of Self-Healing* itemizes twenty attributes (*gunas*), including heaviness, lightness, hotness, coldness, oiliness, dryness, sliminess (viscosity), roughness, liquidity, softness, hardness, cloudiness, and clearness. Furthermore, ayurveda postulates that an "aftertaste" emerges after digestion; that the "aftertaste" of some foods is different from their "taste"; and that, therefore, after assimilation, some foods have an effect (*vipaka*) different from that indicated by their "taste." Finally, the addition of spices or other seasonings to a food supposedly changes its "taste" and, thus, its effect on the *doshas*.

Ayurveda discourages the consumption of foods considered likely to intensify ("aggravate") a particular *dosha* during the season in which that *dosha* predominates. In "Fundamentals of Maharishi Ayur-Veda," Rothenberg stated that, in North America, *vata* predominates from approximately November through February, *kapha* from March through June, and *pitta* from July through October. However, according to *Ayurveda and Immortality* (1986), some ayurvedists hold that *kapha* predominates in winter and that both *kapha* and *pitta* predominate in the spring.

The ayurvedic "diet" is amorphous. In reality, it is a loose framework—composed of empirical and supernaturalistic principles—for selecting, preparing, "combining," and consuming food. For example, in *Perfect Health: The Complete Mind/Body Guide* (1990), Deepak Chopra, M.D., writes:

> A balanced diet does not revolve around fats, carbohydrates, and proteins. Nor are calories, vitamins, and minerals given direct attention. These nutrients are known to us intellectually, not through direct experience. You cannot detect the vitamin C in your orange juice, much less the difference between it and vitamin A. For the most part, Western nutrition comes out of laboratory analysis. Ayurvedic nutrition comes directly from nature. When your taste buds greet a bite of food, an enormous amount of useful information is delivered to the doshas. Working solely with this information, Ayurveda allows us to eat a balanced diet naturally, guided by our own instincts, without turning nutrition into an intellectual headache.

Chopra states that learning one's "body type" is the first step in ayurveda. However, this step is often problematic because "body type" questionnaires differ and because there are ten different "body types": *pitta, kapha, vata,* and seven "combination" types, including *vata-pitta-kapha*. According to Chopra, eating asparagus, okra, chicken, turkey, or shrimp "satisfies," "balances," or "pacifies" all three *doshas*.

The Hindu System of Medicine (1986) states that if diet therapy fails or if the illness is severe, ayurveda recommends fasting, emetics, purgatives, or bloodletting. Indeed, for health maintenance, ayurveda prescribes an emetic biweekly, a purgative every month, and bloodletting twice a year. According to *The Encyclopedia of Eastern Philosophy and Religion* (1989), the "correct conduct of one's life in a religious sense" is "essential" for ayurvedic health maintenance. Traditional ayurvedists treat alcoholism, anorexia, ascites, edema, indigestion, and nausea with a combination of goat feces and urine; constipation with a mixture of milk and urine; impotence with 216 kinds of enemas (some including the testicles of peacocks, swans, and turtles); and epilepsy and insanity with ass urine.

"Spiritual Regeneration" and TM

The Maharishi Mahesh Yogi, founder of transcendental meditation (TM), was born in India in 1911. After attending Allahabad University, he became a monk and for thirteen years studied mysticism in the Himalayas. After his guru's death in 1953, he retreated to a cave, where he lived for two years.

The TM movement began in India in 1955. According to *TM: Discovering Inner Energy and Overcoming Stress* (1975), by Harold H. Bloomfield, M.D., and associates, in 1958 the Maharishi "proclaimed the possibility of all humanity's attaining enlightenment" and inaugurated a "World Plan" intended to encompass "every individual on earth." Shortly thereafter, he embarked upon a world tour to spread his teachings. His world headquarters is now in the Netherlands.

The practice of TM involves sitting in a comfortable position with one's eyes closed for fifteen to twenty minutes in the morning and in the evening. Meditators mentally repeat a mantra—a "secret" magic word that a TM teacher supposedly chooses expressly for the initiate. In contrast, Svoboda states: "A mantra must be pronounced with a particular resonance in a certain area of the body with an appropriate intention and intonation if it is to do any good." According to a pamphlet distributed at a 1993 lecture given by Deepak Chopra, during the practice of TM, "one experiences a unique state of restful alertness which then facilitates the development of one's full creative potential in life."

In the 1970s, sociologist Eric Woodrum investigated the TM movement as a participant and divided it into three phases: During the "Spiritual-Mystical Period" (1959–1965), the Maharishi's Spiritual Regeneration Movement made TM the centerpiece of a "traditional" Hindu program leading ultimately to nirvana—extinction of the ego. During the "Voguish, Self-Sufficiency Period" (1966–1969), the movement assumed a nontraditional and countercultural look, and the goal of nirvana receded. During the "Secularized, Popular-Religious Period," which began in 1970, the movement shifted its public emphasis from "spiritual" goals to the alleged physiological, material, and social benefits of TM for conventional people. It produces a flow of "scientific validation" through an organizational arm, Maharishi International University

(MIU), in Fairfield, Iowa. In early 1993, MIU inaugurated the College of Maharishi Ayur-Ved to offer undergraduate and graduate degrees and a two-month certificate program.

In the mid-1970s, the Maharishi began professing he could teach advanced meditators to levitate. In the Spring 1989 issue of the *Skeptical Inquirer*, Indian magician B. Premanand reported that in 1977 he had challenged the Maharishi to fly by his own power over a distance of about two miles. The Maharishi said he would do so if paid the equivalent of about $1,000, which he believed Premanand and his skeptics group could not afford. However, when they returned the next day with the money, the Maharishi declined to take flight, declaring that TM is not for demonstration purposes. Actually, "yogic flyers" become "airborne" only by hopping and do not reach an altitude of more than a foot.

In 1987, a federal court jury awarded $137,890 to an ex-devotee who contended that TM organizations had falsely promised that he could learn to levitate, reduce stress, improve his memory, and reverse the aging process. In 1988, an appeals court ordered a new trial. On June 20, 1991, the *Des Moines Register* reported that the parties had settled the case out of court for about $50,000.

The National Council Against Health Fraud's March/April 1991 newsletter states: "Paraplegics have been bilked by promises that with enough TM training they would eventually rise from their wheelchairs by levitation." Other alleged benefits of TM and TM-Sidhi (advanced TM) have included elephantine strength, perfect health, immortality, "mastery over nature," "naturally correct" social behavior, and the powers of invisibility, immateriality, and telepathy.

Maharishi Ayur-Ved

"Maharishi Ayur-Ved" is the trade name for the Maharishi Mahesh Yogi's version of ayurveda. Maharishi Ayur-Ved Products International, Inc. (MAPI), defines imbalance as "a build-up or depletion of Vata, Pitta or Kapha (the three mind-body principles) in an individual, beyond the amount natural for his or her mind-body type." In 1985, the Maharishi began marketing a variety of products and services under the trademark "Maharishi Ayur-Veda." MAPI's Autumn/Winter 1993 "Total Health Catalog" includes the following products.

• Maharishi Amrit Kalash (also called "Amrit")—"the cream of Ayurvedic wisdom pressed into form. . . . up to 1,000 times more powerful against free radicals than vitamins C or E." Daily consumption of

Amrit supposedly causes "holistic growth." It consists of two "synergistic and complementary" formulations: Amrit Nectar (or "M4"), a combination of herbs, fruit, ghee and sugar that costs $49.50 for twenty-one ounces; and Ambrosia (or "M5"), herbal tablets that cost 75 cents apiece.

- Maharishi Ayur-Ved Herbals™—"nutrition" supplements that, according to a 1993 flyer, "help restore the proper balance of Vata, Pitta and Kapha in every part of the mind-body system." These "herbals" include *rasayanas*—supposedly time-tested "food supplements" that are "ideal for everyone." Examples of *rasayanas* are: *Rasayana for Students*, which allegedly soothes the brain; *Vital Woman*, which allegedly helps to "harmonize natural rhythms"; *Radiant Skin*, which allegedly nourishes the skin and helps to "bring the beauty from inside out"; *Mind Plus*, which allegedly "nourishes the brain, intellect and nervous system"; and *Meda Formula*, which allegedly helps to "balance and regulate" fat metabolism.

- Teas and seasonings that supposedly help to "balance" *pitta, kapha*, or *vata*

- Sweetened nut-butter spreads with herbs. For example, *Nectar Delight* is a combination of blanched almonds, ghee, whole-milk powder, and Amrit Nectar. MAPI's Autumn/Winter 1993 catalog describes it as a nutritious, healthy, "guilt-free" delicacy and calls ghee "the ideal oil for everyone." *Nectar Delight* costs $4.95 for four ounces. A January 1994 mailing described another spread, *Almond Delight*, as "especially good for Vata, because the herbs nourish the mind while the almonds give a wholesome burst of energy."

- Aromatherapy oils that supposedly help to "reconnect" mind and body

- Shampoos and massage oils labeled "pitta," "vata," or "kapha"

- Vedic music cassettes and compact discs that MAPI says should be selected for play according to the time of day or night

- Audiotapes of "historic" lectures by the Maharishi

According to "The Total Health Catalog," the Ayur-Ved system of "natural health care" includes the following approaches.

- TM and TM-Sidhi

- Primordial sound therapy, which allegedly uses "the frequencies of natural law structured in the consciousness of every individual" to "restore balance in the individual and society" (Mentally repeating the Sanskrit word *"amrita,"* which means "nectar of immortality," constitutes the "primordial sound" approach.)

• *Gandharva-Ved* therapy, the use of Vedic music "to restore physiological balance in the individual and nature as a whole"

• *Panchakarma* (see below)

• *Rasayana* therapy, the use of ayurvedic herbal preparations (see above)

• Pulse reading—"to identify any existing or future imbalance and to indicate the necessary treatment programs to restore and maintain perfect health"

• Maharishi *jyotish*, a "mathematical approach to understanding the basis of maintaining balance, including procedures to identify the exact timing and nature of future imbalances along with the precautions necessary to avert the danger before it arises" (i.e., Hindu astrology)

• Maharishi *yagya*, a set of "procedures to promote balance in the individual and the community and bring the support of natural law to daily life" (i.e., ceremonies aimed at winning the blessings of Hindu deities)

In *Perfect Health*, Chopra defines *panchakarma* as "purification treatment." The goal of *panchakarma* is to rid the body of *ama* ("residual impurities deposited in the cells as the result of improper digestion"). Chopra lists six steps of *panchakarma*: (1) "oleation," the ingestion of clarified butter or a medicated oil "to soften up the doshas and minimize digestive action"; (2) administration of a laxative to reduce *pitta*; (3) oil massage, with oil "herbalized" according to constitutional type; (4) "herbalized" steam treatments; (5) administration of medicated enemas (ayurveda "lists well over a hundred") to "flush the loosened doshas out through the intestinal tract"; and (6) "inhalation" of medicinal oils or herbal mixtures.

"Maharishi Ayur-Ved: Approaches to the Prevention of Disease and the Promotion of Perfect Health," a booklet published in 1993 by the Maharishi Ayur-Ved Medical Association, quotes the Maharishi: "Through the introduction of Ayur-Ved it is completely within the ability of any government or its responsible, eminent people to create a disease-free society and enjoy perfect health, continued progress, self-sufficiency, and invincibility." In 1992, proponents launched the Natural Law Party and fielded a presidential candidate and many candidates for state and federal offices. A twenty-four-page advertisement, in tabloid format, expressed its platform. The health section stated:

> The Natural Law Party envisions a disease-free society, in which every American enjoys a long life in perfect health. By bringing life into accord with natural law, the prevention programs proposed by the Natural Law Party will eliminate disease and culture ideal health and vitality for everyone. . . .
> Research suggests that implementing the programs proposed by the Natural Law Party could cut healthcare costs in half, saving an estimated $400 billion annually for the nation.

However, consider the following request from transcendental meditators. In November 1989, TM leaders in the Washington, D.C., area circulated a letter throughout the TM community that solicited donations for the ayurvedic "treatment" of a member allegedly suffering from "rectal endometriosis." They described this as a potentially fatal illness involving "abnormal tissue growth in the lining and/or outer surface of the abdominal organs" and conveyed an ayurvedic physician's "primary recommendation": the patient should *"receive a Yagya as soon as possible."* Reportedly, the "recommended amount needed" for the patient's "recovery"—*minus* "basic living expenses" (which included an inexplicit "program fee")—was $34,600 *per year.* The "recommended amount needed" for the *yagya* was $11,600; the "less than recommended" amount was $8,500; and the minimal amount was $3,300.

The Mystical Medic of Never-Never Land

Deepak Chopra, M.D., was born and raised in New Delhi, India, and attended the All India Institute of Medical Sciences. After graduation, he moved to the United States and completed residencies in internal medicine and endocrinology. According to a 1993 lecture pamphlet, after becoming chief of staff at the New England Memorial Hospital and establishing a large private practice, Chopra "noticed a growing lack of fulfillment and the nagging question, 'Am I doing all I can for my patients?'" These problems, the pamphlet states, inspired him to learn TM and meet the Maharishi. The May/June 1990 issue of *In Health* relates that after meeting Chopra in 1985, the Maharishi persuaded him to found the American Association of Ayurvedic Medicine and become medical director of the Maharishi Ayur-Veda Health Center for Behavioral Medicine and Stress Management in Lancaster, Massachusetts.

In 1993, I received several mailings from Nightingale-Conant Corporation, near Chicago, which markets audiocassette programs. These include

Chopra's "Magical Mind, Magical Body," "The Higher Self," and "Weight Loss—The Complete Mind/Body Approach." One of the six "Magical Mind" cassettes, titled "You Are the Universe," invites the listener "to become a citizen of the cosmos." The "Magical Mind" mailing included a "personal message" from Chopra that describes his first meeting with the Maharishi:

> When I was back in India on vacation, I was open to all points of view. And when Maharishi Mahesh Yogi . . . asked me to see him, I went. He said very simply, "I have been waiting a long time to bring out some special techniques. I believe they will become the medicine of the future. They were known in the distant past, but were lost in the confusion of time. I want you to learn them, and then to explain clearly and scientifically how they work." I listened. I took notes. On my return home to Boston, I tried these techniques in my personal life. I can't begin to tell you how much better I felt, how vigorous, how young! Soon I began to tell patients about it—and then to see the most amazing results!

The "Higher Self" mailing included another message from Chopra, which describes the "higher self" as "an infinite reservoir of intelligence" and "the living force that knows why you are here on earth, what you need and how to get it." In this message, Chopra claims that "spiritual needs for love, compassion, meaningfulness, total acceptance and inner peace" are "fulfilled spontaneously" when one finds one's "Higher Self." He also states:

> You *are* your own reality.
> You create it; you carry it around with you; and, most importantly, you project it onto everyone else and everything else you encounter.
> But the traditional Western notion of reality is much too limiting for a true realization of life. If you are to understand yourself and the world around you properly, you need to expand your boundaries of reality—of time, space and matter.
> Once you've done this, you can align the energy of your physical body with the energy of the universe.

An advertisement in the August 1993 issue of *Body, Mind & Spirit* suggests that Chopra's "Weight Loss" program enables people to "literally change" their bodies as easily as they change their clothes—"*without* diets or deprivation!" In the same issue, Nina L. Diamond quotes Chopra: "The [research] methodology is different in Alternative Medicine. We have to include things like the patient's relationship with the doctor, the flow of consciousness between the two." She further quotes him: "In a few years every hospital will have an Alternative Medicine section. And every medical school will have [an] alternative department."

Chopra was a keynote speaker at Newlife Expo '93, held at the Hotel Ramada in New York City, which I attended on April 24. Others scheduled to give lectures or conduct workshops included proponents of acupuncture, aikido, aromatherapy, astrology, aura balancing, bioenergetics, the cabala, channeling, crystal healing, "essence repatterning," Gerson therapy, guided meditation, herbalism, homeopathy, Huna, iridology, kundalini yoga, magic, numerology, past-life therapy, Qigong, rebirthing, reflexology, reiki, shiatsu, tai chi, tantra, the tarot, healing "through the human voice," plant-enzyme "shortcuts" to health, communication with "nature spirits," "living foods for self-healing," *The Urantia Book* (a bible reputedly authored by a committee of superhuman extraterrestrials), and body harmony (a "hands-on" healing technique that allegedly "reawakens" one's "natural healing energies"). Exhibitors included Charlotte Gerson, president of the Gerson Institute; the Church of Universal Knowledge; the Egyptian Mystery School; a company marketing products supposedly imbued with "tachyon energy"; an institute promoting a "non-invasive" manual technique "empowered by universal energy"; and proponents of African holistic health, aura analysis, chiropractic, cranial balancing, holistic dentistry, macrobiotics, Natural Hygiene, polarity therapy, psychic surgery, reiki, and cymatics ("the healing nature of sound"). The organizers devoted one large room to counseling by psychics for hire, and another large room to such bodywork methods as the Alexander technique, the hakomi method, reflexology, reiki, and rolfing. Admission to the health fair was $10. Attendance at Chopra's lecture cost an additional $25. At the fair, I also spent about $6.50 on a lunch of beans, carrots, noodles, tofu "cutlets"—all cold and oily—and a "leaden" dessert.

In the grand ballroom, the site of Chopra's lecture, a pamphlet published by Quantum Publications in South Lancaster, Massachusetts, lay on each seat. It featured a piece by Chopra titled "The Value of Innocence," wherein he bemoans the "banishment" of innocence to "Peter Pan's Never-Never Land." He defines innocence as "living in complete contact with your higher self, trusting it to guide you all the time"; and he advocates a "simple, open, trusting life." Chopra, who looked overweight, was eloquent, urbane, and charming—an erudite crowdpleaser. *Newlife* magazine editor-publisher Mark Becker introduced him as an expert who can reach the public.

Chopra stated that the aim of his lecture was to introduce briefly the subject matter of his new book, *Ageless Body, Timeless Mind: The Quantum Alternative To Growing Old* (1993). He intimated that he was 150 years old:

> We have a lot of mythology about what is supposed to be normal aging. What we call normal aging in our society is actually the psychopathology of the average. One thing that [Mark Becker] didn't do when he

was introducing me is tell you that I'm a hundred and fifty years old. What we call "aging normally" in our society is probably the result of the hypnosis of social conditioning—an induced fiction that we have selectively agreed to participate in.

Chopra further stated:

The spirit . . . is a real force. Until now, science has sort of shied away from talking about the spirit. . . . Science, until recently, has not addressed the crucial question, "What is this thing that is known as the spirit?" The spirit is a real force. It's as real as gravity or time. It's equally as abstract, equally as incomprehensible, equally as mysterious, but much, much more powerful. If you get in touch with that innermost core of your being, you're getting in touch with the core of what life is, its most basic core. Life is nothing other than spirit in disguise.

Chopra outlined what he called the "ten characteristics of the experience of active mastery." These include: recognition that "the body, the flesh, is not really separate from the spirit"; renouncement of the "need for judgment"; and perception of the universe and all experience as a "projection" or "reflection" of oneself, of who one is. "The presence of God is everywhere," he said. "The reason most people are unable to have the experience [of active mastery] . . . is that their entire reality is based on a superstition . . . the superstition of materialism, which holds. . . that this is a material world, that we are material bodies, that we are separate from each other in space and time." "Life," he restated, "is in its most essential form . . . the spirit." Chopra contended that the "superstition of materialism" describes the human body as "a frozen anatomical structure, a physical machine." He said the body is actually: "a river of intelligence, of energy, and of information"; "merely recycled earth, water, and air"; a "field of ideas." He claimed that all body cells are "conscious little beings" that have thoughts, memories, emotions, and desire. He explained: "When you say, 'My heart is heavy with sadness,' your heart is loaded with sad chemicals. When you say, 'I'm bursting with joy,' your skin is loaded with happy molecules." He later stated:

Your mind is not in your body. . . . Your body is in your mind, and your mind is in something else . . . the spirit. . . . The body is the objective experience of consciousness, the mind is the subjective experience of consciousness, but consciousness is the only reality.

In Part Four of *Ageless Body, Timeless Mind*, Chopra states: "Depleted Prana is directly linked to aging and death. Nothing can remain alive when Prana is absent." He then puts forth "rules" to "ensure" the conservation of *prana*. These involve consumption of fresh produce (preferably homegrown) and pure water, sunning, moderate exercise, slow and regular breathing, peaceful ("life-nourishing") behavior, and "positive emotions, particularly love." Yet in Part Five, he claims that death is an illusion "based on a very selective view of reality that was conditioned into you before you had a conscious choice." He states: "Death isn't a brute fact but a mystery, and it must be unraveled before the mystery of aging—the process that leads to death—can be solved."

"That's the Spirit"

On July 12, 1993, Chopra was the sole guest on Oprah Winfrey's talk show. The ABC telecast centered on *Ageless Body, Timeless Mind.* Winfrey said she had decided to interview Chopra on her show after singer Michael Jackson had phoned her from Chopra's house and demanded his appearance. She stated that Jackson was a "special friend" of Chopra's. Winfrey asked Chopra to "talk about how we're all connected—mind, body, and spirit." Chopra responded:

> The mind is the thought that we have. The body is the molecules—the chemicals—that those thoughts produce. But who is having those thoughts? That's the spirit. And the spirit is in the silent spaces between the thoughts. . . .
> In every little space between my thoughts is the infinite choice-maker. That's the spirit.

Later he stated: "If you really want to heal yourself, then you want to get in touch with that part of yourself that's not time-bound, that's not in the field of change, that's nonchanging. . . . That part of you that doesn't change is the spirit." On her October 18, 1993 program, which featured neospiritualist Raymond Moody, M.D., Winfrey, an avowed theist, said she regarded bodies as "outfits" and human beings as spirits "inside some flesh and bones." This program focused on a chamber or "scrying room" Moody had built in his house. The design of this room supposedly facilitates communication, or a "healing" reunion, with deceased persons. ABC rebroadcast both programs in December 1993.

In an interview in the July 8, 1993 issue of *The San Diego Union-Tribune*, Chopra stated that he had dissociated himself from organizations that advocate the Maharishi or TM but said he still recommends TM. In a letter to "friends," he stated that shortly after deciding to terminate his position of leadership within the TM movement, he was hired by Sharp HealthCare, a large group of hospitals in San Diego, to set up and direct the Institute for Human Potential and Mind

Body Medicine. The program, he said, would include ayurvedic medicine but would be open to other modes of therapy. Although his letter said he would continue to support the movement, a Maharishi National Council member advised other Maharishi Ayur-Ved leaders to stop promoting Chopra, his lectures, and his publications.

"A Negative Approach to Human Existence"

In *Mental Alchemy* (1984), Rosicrucian "imperator" Ralph M. Lewis, an advocate of meditation, criticized TM and yoga philosophy in general:

> Transcendental meditation from the psychological point of view is a loss of personal identity with the reality of our world. It is the attempt to enter into a wholly subjective state for full realization of reality. . . . Further, [TM] should not be used as an escape from the world of reality as it is so commonly done by devotees . . . . It is true that what reality is we do not actually know. We receive only impressions of it through our receptor senses. These are transformed into sensations which we interpret. However, our physical existence is dependent upon our adjustment to such illusions—if that is what they are. . . .
>
> To consider the body a prison of self, something to be demeaned, and to think of the appetites and passions as being that which should be completely suppressed is a *false* conception.
>
> We should not endeavor to escape the world and its impact on our life but rather to *master* our personal life in this world. . . . To endeavor to live in a mental and psychic vacuum through any method is a negative approach to human existence.

Urine Therapy

Urine therapy is a "remedy" with Hindu roots wherein the patient's urine is ingested, injected, introduced into the rectum, and/or used topically. Hindus credit urine with "purifying powers" and regard urine from cows as a "sacred cleanser." In the 1970s, a former Indian prime minister stated on American television that he drank some of his own urine daily for health maintenance. He called urine "the water of life." Contemporary Western proponents of urine therapy claim it can cure acne, AIDS, arthritis, chronic fatigue syndrome, herpes, and leprosy. In *The Miracles of Urine-Therapy* (1987), naturopathic chiropractor Beatrice Bartnett and licensed massage therapist Margie Adelman extol urine as the blood of Christ, the fountain of youth, and "a gift given by your creator for your spiritual growth and physical well-being." Bartnett and Adelman recommend that people drink their own urine to "cleanse" the body of "toxins." They list several side effects: nausea, vomiting, migraines, boils, pimples, rashes, palpitations, diarrhea, uneasiness, and fever. However, they emphasize that these side effects are "NORMAL" and that patients should not fear them. In a "special section" on AIDS, they state:

> AIDS will AID us in bringing about change.... AIDS provides great hope and a chance for a spiritual revolution which will establish peace on earth! AIDS is truly the miracle of the twentieth century!

"Believe in the power of the God energy," they advise, "and you will find it exists *within* your vehicle."

If ayurveda seems "quaintly newfangled," macrobiotics—the subject of the following chapter—appears to be wearing thin.

6

Macrobiotics

Macrobiotics is a quasireligious movement and "antidisease" lifestyle founded by George Ohsawa (1893–1966) and popularized in the United States by Michio Kushi. Its centerpiece is a diet that emphasizes grains and discourages consumption of animal foods. The thrust of macrobiotic nutrition is not to optimize nutrient intake but to regulate two alleged elementary forms of energy: yin and yang. Assignment of "yin-ness" and "yang-ness" to foods is based largely on characteristics directly perceptible by the senses and is unrelated to nutrient composition.

Zen Macrobiotics

Advocates of the earliest version of the diet, called the "Zen macrobiotic diet," claimed it could cure numerous and disparate health problems, including airsickness, bedwetting, cataracts, retinal detachment, nearsightedness, epilepsy, baldness, gonorrhea, syphilis, hemophilia, leprosy, polio, and schizophrenia. Proponents ascribed all these conditions to a dietary imbalance of yin and yang. In *Zen Macrobiotics* (1965), Ohsawa wrote that dandruff is "the first step toward mental disease" and that leprosy, "like cancer . . . is very easy to cure," attacking "only those with a very good constitution by birth."

The Zen macrobiotic diet involved seven classes of food and ten progressively restrictive dietary stages, termed "ways to health and happiness." The lowest stage comprised 10 percent grains, 30 percent vegetables, 10 percent soup, 30 percent animal products, 15 percent fruits and salads, and 5 percent desserts. Each "higher" (supposedly more healthful) stage called for 10 percent more grains and progressively less "animal" and "salad/fruit" items. The fourth stage eliminated fruits, the sixth stage all animal products, and the "highest" stage everything except grains. Ohsawa discouraged fluid intake at all stages.

In 1966, a Passaic (New Jersey) grand jury reviewed three cases of death and two cases of near-death from malnutrition among Zen macrobiotic adherents. The jury concluded that the diet "constitutes a public health hazard." In 1967, the *Journal of the American Medical Association* reported how one of these adherents had developed scurvy within ten months of starting the diet. These cases set the tone for scientific medicine's view of macrobiotics. In 1971, the AMA Council on Foods and Nutrition stated that followers of the diet, particularly the highest level, stood in "great danger" of malnutrition.

In *Macrobiotics: Yesterday and Today* (1985), macrobiotics insider Ronald E. Kotzsch, Ph.D., describes how Beth Ann Simon, a young New Yorker, followed the diet's highest stage and died in 1965—apparently of malnutrition and dehydration. Her death eventuated in a lawsuit against Ohsawa for malpractice and the closing of the Ohsawa Foundation in New York. The hub of macrobiotics on the East Coast then shifted to Boston and its resident Ohsawa disciple, Michio Kushi.

The Kushi Era

Michio Kushi was born in Japan in 1926 and studied political science and international law before coming to the United States in 1949. In 1965, he moved from New York to Cambridge, Massachusetts, and founded the Erewhon Trading Company. The company operated a small basement retail outlet for macrobiotic foods in nearby Boston. "Erewhon" is both the title of a utopian novel by Victorian satirist Samuel Butler and the name of Ohsawa's metaphor for a model Japan. In *Zen Macrobiotics*, Ohsawa asserted that "Erewhon" is "nowhere" spelled backwards. Kushi's store grossed about $200 to $300 weekly in 1967. However, as attendance at macrobiotic lectures increased, the business expanded into "nonmacrobiotic" foods (such as dairy products and honey) and "organically grown" foods. By the time it filed for bankruptcy in 1981, Erewhon encompassed more than ten stores, a large wholesale warehouse, and a macrobiotic rural community called Erewhon Farms.

In the 1970s, Kushi helped organize *East West Journal*, the East West Foundation, and the Kushi Institute. In 1981, the Kushi Foundation was established as the parent organization for the institute and the magazine. A few years later, One Peaceful World—a society dedicated to "planetary health"—

was formed under the aegis of the foundation. *East West* was sold to outside investors in 1989, was renamed *East West Natural Health* in 1992, and is now called *Natural Health*.

The Kushi Institute occupies six hundred acres in Becket, Massachusetts. Besides holding lectures, seminars, and conferences, the institute markets more than a hundred books, audiocassettes, and videotapes about macrobiotics and other topics consistent with its beliefs. There are affiliated institutes in Amsterdam, Antwerp, Barcelona, Florence, Lisbon, London, and Kiental (Switzerland) and about six hundred independent macrobiotic "centers" in many parts of the world. The institute reportedly has provided thousands of people with instruction in macrobiotic principles and techniques. Its Leadership Studies Program has extension programs in several American cities. It comprises three five-week tiers, each focused on personal, societal, or planetary health. Core subjects include Oriental diagnosis and *ki* development ("energy adjustment"). The total cost of the program is $8,250. In November 1993, a telephone receptionist told me that "Kushi House"—Kushi's residence in Brookline, the Boston suburb that had hosted the institute's headquarters between 1977 and 1992—was "part of the Kushi Institute" and a site for "consultations."

Natural Health, published bimonthly, contains about a hundred and fifty pages per issue and has a circulation of about 175,000. Its editorial philosophy is leery of scientific medicine and supportive of vitalistic systems and methods, including: acupuncture, homeopathy, kundalini meditation, naturopathy, past-life therapy, and rolfing. Products that typify advertisements in *Natural Health* include: an "oxygen supplement" (supposedly furnishing vitamin "O"), a "multivitamin skin cream" ("the perfect skin food"), "guided imagery" audiotapes for cancer and AIDS, "music composed in a trance," an "elemental diode" that allegedly shields its wearer from electromagnetic fields, Vedic horoscopes, and an "improved" remedy for thinning hair available by mail for $93.

What is Macrobiotics?

The word "macrobiotics" derives from two Greek words: *makros*, meaning "large," and *biotos*, meaning "life." A Kushi Foundation pamphlet translates these Greek words as "great life." In *Zen Macrobiotics*, Ohsawa called macrobiotics "the medicine of longevity and rejuvenation." *Webster's Dictionary* defines macrobiotics as "the art of prolonging life." *The New Age Dictionary* (1990)—edited by Alex Jack, former editor-in-chief of *East West*— includes a definition ascribed to Michio Kushi:

the way of health, happiness, and peace through biological and spiritual evolution and the universal means to practice and harmonize with the Order of the Universe in daily life, including the selection, preparation, and manner of cooking and eating, as well as the orientation of consciousness toward infinite spiritual realization.

However, Ronald Kotzsch observed: "There is no explicit, generally accepted understanding of what it means to be 'macrobiotic.' Macrobiotics is many-faceted. It includes a diet, a system of medicine, a philosophy, a way of life, a community, and a broad social movement." And in the April/May 1990 issue of *To Your Health* ("The Magazine of Healing and Hope"), Asher Lazar called the term "macrobiotics" a misnomer and opined that the word "traditionalism" better characterizes the aims of macrobiotics.

Macrobiotics attributes many of its ideas to traditional Chinese medicine. According to ancient Chinese cosmology, yin and yang are the opposite but complementary cosmic principles or "energy modes" that compose the *tao*. The word "*tao*" derives from a Mandarin word meaning "way"; it stands for ultimate reality, universal energy, and living in harmony with the universe. *Tao: To Know and Not Be Knowing* (1993) states:

> The Tao is an experience rather than a "thought." It is essentially too comprehensive and all-embracing simply to be understood through a single mental expression, and is therefore difficult for the Western mind to interpret. It is . . . the essential reality from which all resulting ways may be understood. . . . In order to recognize the Law of Tao within and outside of ourselves . . . the individual must abandon all ideas that have been imposed from the outside and return instead to the original nature.

Taoists hold that unadulterated human nature is a reflection of the nature of the universe and therefore merits following. The *tao* is thus analogous to the "natural laws" of so-called natural healing (see Chapter 8).

In Chinese tradition, the sky (the generator of all phenomena) exemplifies yang, the active, bright, male principle, while the earth exemplifies yin, the passive, dark, female principle. Macrobiotics cites yin-yang theory and categorizes phenomena and ideas as either yin or yang. However, while the Chinese theory (which includes acupuncture) distinguishes by function, macrobiotics distinguishes according to structure. For example, macrobiotics categorizes the earth as yang because it is denser than the sky (that is, the rest of the universe); Chinese cosmology takes the opposite view. According to the eighth edition of Ohsawa's *Philosophy of Oriental Medicine*:

> In old Chinese medicine, the small intestine, bladder, stomach, large intestine, etc., are classified as yang while the heart, kidneys, pancreas,

liver, etc., are classified as yin. This is a *metaphysical classification*. Physically speaking, this must be reversed: all empty organs are yin, as they are passive and receptive; all solid organs, with density and compactness, are yang.

A Kushi Foundation pamphlet states: "Macrobiotics is understanding the energetics of food and how to make the choices which can lead you in a more centered and positive direction. . . . As your body and mind become healthier and clearer, you will joyfully realize the boundless energy that lies within us all." Macrobiotic assignment of "yin-ness" or "yang-ness" to foods is based on factors distant from nutrient composition. Theoretically, these include the region and season of the food's cultivation and its color, pH, shape, size, taste, temperature, texture, water content, and weight. The manner of preparation and consumption also affects the "yin/yang-ness" of foods.

In *Zen Macrobiotics*, Ohsawa advised that "principal food"—cereals (grains), sautéed vegetables, and soup—constitutes at least 60 percent of one's diet. Taken out of context, this recommendation does not sound unreasonable. However, he further advised consuming foods within his seven classes that are at or "reasonably near" the midpoint of yin and yang—"unless there is a *specific* reason for another choice." Ohsawa's "reasons" included schizophrenia (a "yin disease" for which he recommended "all yang drinks") and kidney disease in general (for which he recommended brown-rice juice and azuki-bean juice with a pinch of salt). Moreover, several pages later Ohsawa defined "principal foods" as "only" cereals.

Yin-yang theory, Eastern religious underpinnings, and a Japanese culinary bias make macrobiotics intriguing to many Westerners. However, its diet is reducible to the consumption of unprocessed or minimally processed foods, primarily whole grains and vegetables, which, ideally, should be grown "organically" in the region where the consumer lives and eaten in season. Kushi advises chewing food slowly and quietly at least fifty times per mouthful or until it liquefies. His "standard macrobiotic diet"—designed primarily for residents of temperate regions—encompasses the following.

- Cooked, "organically grown," whole grains—an average of 50 percent of the volume of each meal

- Soup made with vegetables, seaweed, grains, or beans, usually seasoned with miso or soy sauce—about 5 to 10 percent of daily food intake

- "Organic" vegetables, preferably grown locally, mostly cooked—about 20 to 30 percent of daily food intake

- Cooked beans, soybean-based products, and seaweed—about 5 to 10 percent of daily food intake

- Beverages: "traditional," nonstimulating, non-aromatic teas (such as roasted brown rice tea); and water—preferably spring water or "quality" well water—not iced, and in moderation

- Fresh, white-meat fish—5 to 15 percent of food intake on one to three days each week, "if needed or desired"

- Fresh, dried, and cooked fruit, preferably grown locally and "organically"—two or three servings per week

- Occasional snacks: lightly roasted nuts, peanuts, and seeds

- Condiments: unrefined sesame oil, unrefined corn oil from stone-ground corn, sea salt, soy sauce, miso, gomashio (a mixture of dry-roasted and crushed sesame seeds and sea salt), seaweed powder, pickles such as umeboshi (a Japanese plum), tekka (a mixture of minced lotus root, burdock root, carrot, ginger, and miso), and sauerkraut.

Foods "to avoid for better health" include meat, poultry, dairy products, refined sugars, molasses, honey, vanilla, tropical and semitropical fruits and fruit juices, coffee, mint teas, potatoes, sweet potatoes, yams, tomatoes, eggplant, peppers, asparagus, spinach, avocado, hot spices, refined grains, and all canned, frozen, or irradiated foods. Proponents discourage nutritional supplementation, and fluid restriction is common. Kushi has adapted his "standard diet" to over twenty types of cancer. In his column in the Late Summer 1993 issue of *MacroNews*, he states:

> Cancer . . . is not an enemy, but a friend. . . . Cancer is the body's own defense mechanism to protect itself against long-term dietary and environmental abuse. Cancer cells are localizing toxins in our body, allowing it to continue functioning until fundamental changes in diet and lifestyle are made. Cancer cells are working in harmony with all other cells. . . . This is an example of the natural attraction and harmony that is found throughout the universe.

In the January 1986 issue of *Health Foods Business*, Rebecca Theurer Wood offered advice to managers of health-food stores:

> Let's look at what turns an otherwise normal human being into a macrobiotic. In understanding this, we might better serve and/or help create the macrobiotic clientele.

The majority of people who start macrobiotics today suffer from a degenerative illness and are attempting to cure themselves. They've read some macrobiotic literature . . . or have had a consultation from one of Michio Kushi's students. They come into your store with a grocery list of macrobiotics supplies to purchase.

For most, it's their maiden venture into a natural foods store, and they'll buy strange items that they've never even heard of—let alone can pronounce or cook. In other words, they're overwhelmed.

Have your employees watch for such shoppers whose lists include miso and umeboshi. Help cushion their first experience in your store by extending personable service. . . . Assure these neophytes that macrobiotic staples are edible and that sea vegetables are actually delicious. Point out some of your staff who eat this way. Better yet, name drop macrobiotic superstars such as John Denver or Dirk Benedict. . . .

Work with the macrobiotic center or counselor nearest your area. . . . Refer people to him/her. He'll/she'll certainly be sending customers to you. Sponsor macrobiotic lectures and cooking classes. Post the counselor's calendar and business card.

"Other Dimensions"

Macrobiotics embraces a plethora of supernatural beliefs. (As a Kushi Foundation pamphlet states, "Macrobiotics is more than a hill of beans.") Besides liberalizing Ohsawa's diet, Kushi expanded and "paranormalized" Ohsawa's already supernaturalistic philosophy, merging into the macrobiotic mainstream such matters as: chanting, creative visualization, dream interpretation, Japanese astrology ("nine star ki"), karma, oriental physiognomy (including "diagnosis" of beauty marks), palmistry, shiatsu, ghosts, the "macrobiotic lifestyle" of Jesus Christ and his disciples, extraterrestrial encounters, exploring unexplained "other dimensions," and "seeing harmony in dualism." In the introduction to *Standard Macrobiotic Diet* (1992), Kushi states: "The goal of macrobiotics is to preserve the human race and to create a new species—*homo spiritus.*" One of his "timeless and universal" teachings is that a depressed navel indicates a yang constitution and a protuberant navel symptomizes a yin constitution. The latter, Kushi says, may be the result of excessive fluid intake by one's mother during pregnancy.

The "diagnostic" methods espoused by Kushi are alien to scientific medicine. They are part of what he calls natural medicine, which he defines as "the medicine of energy and vibrations." In *Your Face Never Lies: An*

Introduction to Oriental Diagnosis (1983), Kushi equated *ki* with *chi*, *prana*, and orgone. He claimed that facial lines and wrinkles and skin discolorations indicate the condition of internal organs. According to Kushi, horizontal lines on the forehead and below the eyes manifest excessive intake of sugars, fats, and liquid; long, thick eyebrows signify happiness and vitality and portend longevity; a swollen nose indicates that the heart is swollen; and a swollen lower lip indicates a tendency to constipation.

In *The Macrobiotic Approach to Cancer* (1991), he advocates a form of sclerology, claiming that: (1) tiny dark spots in the upper half of the white portion of the eyeball often indicate the formation of calcified deposits in the sinuses; (2) dark spots in the lower half often indicate the formation of kidney stones and may also indicate ovarian cysts; (3) a blue, green, or brown discoloration—or "white patches"—near the left or right side of the iris often indicates the accumulation of mucus and fat in the liver, gallbladder, spleen, and pancreas; and (4) a yellow discoloration of the lower part of the eye often indicates accumulation of fat and mucus in and around the prostate or in the female sex organs, and it may also indicate vaginal discharges, ovarian cysts, fibroid tumors, and other gynecological disorders.

In the Spring 1993 issue of *MacroNews*, Kushi describes *rei-so*, or spiritual diagnosis, as a type of Oriental diagnosis based on "seeing the influences exerted by people who have died." He states:

> Wandering spirits appear over the shoulders. If they appear over the left shoulder, they are either male spirits . . . or are among the father's ancestors. If they appear over the right shoulder, they are either female spirits or are of the mother's ancestors. Spirits that are influencing us negatively create darkness in our aura . . . .
>
> Our health may depend on whether we can make our spiritual condition clean and clear by pacifying and releasing any attached spirits. Prayer, self-reflection, and changing the quality of our blood cells and entire being through a balanced natural diet are necessary to achieve this.

According to the macrobiotic "way of life," one should: feel grateful toward nature and one's ancestors; walk barefoot daily, in simple clothing, on grass, soil, or the beach; use only "natural" and "organic" cosmetics; minimize the use of color televisions and computers; and sing a happy song every day. Moreover, one should refrain from: wearing synthetic clothing directly on the skin (it supposedly interferes with the body's "energy flow"); taking a long, hot bath or shower unless one has consumed too much salt or animal food; and using electrical cooking appliances.

Kushi glorified his revision of macrobiotics in an early 1994 issue of *MacroNews*:

What we presently call "macrobiotics" is the first biological revolution to occur since the appearance of homo sapiens on this planet. With the exception of a few rare individuals, humanity has only been following heaven and earth, and has been subject to natural evolution and natural degeneration. From now on, we can choose to develop ourselves or make ourselves decline. . . . That is the meaning of the tree of life prophesied in the Bible. Until now we have had ample opportunity to eat from the tree of knowledge, but have yet to eat from the tree of life. That era is now coming. After millions of years on the planet, humanity has finally come of age. Friends who are eating whole grains and vegetables and studying the principles of life are like the early pioneers. In the future, their way of life will guide humanity toward one peaceful world.

Mission to "Mecca"

Before 1988, macrobiotics had merely puzzled me, but during my existential crisis its mystique prompted me to read about ten books on the subject. In that year, several occupational factors combined with my penchant for mystical and occult literature to spur my investigation of "paranormal nutrition." At the time, I worked as a clinical dietitian in a hospital that served a poor community. The paperwork was repetitive and extensive, leaving time only for cursory nutritional counseling. Three of my four dietitian coworkers were obese and one was overweight. In contrast, macrobiotics spotlighted dietary treatment and education and its practitioners seemed to practice what they preached.

After reading Kotzsch's *Macrobiotics: Yesterday and Today* with fascination, I wrote to Stephen Barrett, M.D., then editor of *Nutrition Forum* newsletter, and proposed my attending a program at the Kushi Institute and writing an article about it.. Although Dr. Barrett assumed that I was intent on discrediting macrobiotics, I was actually sympathetic to what I considered "dissident dietetics." The newsletter subsidized my attendance at the Michio Kushi Seminar for Medical Professionals, held from June 20 to June 25, 1989. The eighteen other participants included twelve medical doctors, two registered nurses, and an osteopath.

During the seminar, Kushi purportedly demonstrated the existence of chakras. He held a thread with nail clippers attached to its lower end over two attendees. In both cases, the nail clippers moved in a circle. Kushi claimed that chakras caused this movement, but I noticed that his arm also moved. Between lectures, two doctors tried to duplicate Kushi's "demonstration." When I told the one holding the nail clippers that her arm was moving, she invited me to try. I did so, keeping my arm still, and the nail clippers did not move. Apparently undaunted, the doctor responded: "Oh, my God, when somebody wants to, they can really botch this."

All attendees received an information packet that contained descriptions of thirteen categories of "diagnosis" Kushi allegedly has used. I have paraphrased the descriptions for clarity:

- *Visual diagnosis:* Observing all visible characteristics of the human body to discover "any major internal disorders" in certain systems, functions, organs, or glands

- *Pulse diagnosis:* Examining the pulse at both wrists, the neck, the feet, and other areas to detect "physical or psychological details"

- *Meridian diagnosis:* Inspecting meridians (longitudinal lines representing alleged channels for chi) for colors and spots, which supposedly provide "valuable information" on "internal energy flow," organ function, and other metabolic activity

- *Pressure diagnosis:* Applying pressure to more than a hundred areas on the body to reveal "any stagnation of the streaming energy in the circulatory and nervous functions related to physical and psychological conditions"

- *Voice diagnosis:* Listening to various forms of vocal communication to identify disorders of certain systems, organs, or glands

- *Behavioral diagnosis:* Observing behaviors, manners, motions, or patterns of movement to identify psychological, physical, and dietary problems

- *Psychological diagnosis:* Observing behavior, dreams, speech, "ways of thinking," and other "expressions" to reveal psychological status—especially to determine which parts of the brain and nervous system are "actively stimulated" or "negatively understimulated"

- *Astrological diagnosis:* Considering the time and place of birth, the place where the subject was raised, current place of residence, and current astrological and astronomical conditions to characterize basic physical and mental tendencies and the potential destiny of the subject in this life and a "future life"

- *Environmental diagnosis:* Considering temperature, humidity, "celestial influences," tidal motions, seasonal conditions, and residential and occupational conditions to determine the "environmental cause" of physical and psychological disorders

- *Parental and ancestral diagnosis:* Using visual diagnosis (see above) and considering the lifestyle of the subject's parents and ancestors to reveal hereditary physical and psychological tendencies and to predict the subject's future

- *Aura and vibrational diagnosis:* Accurately appraising the subject's "aura" and "vibrations" in terms of intensity, color, temperature, and frequency—without any instrument—to understand the subject's "comprehensive" physical and psychological condition

- *Consciousness and thought diagnosis:* Observing behavior, "expression," and the patterns of vibrations emanating from the head to read the subject's mind

- *Spiritual diagnosis:* Evaluating "atmospheric vibrational conditions" to identify "spiritual influences," including memories and "visions of the future"

When I last saw Kushi at the seminar, he exhorted the physicians to fulfill their true role as teachers of the macrobiotic way of life.

The Bottom Line

Researchers have reported serious health problems due to dietary deficiency resulting from adherence to a restrictive macrobiotic diet. The diet's reputation for curing cancer rests merely on testimonials from patients—many of whom received conventional treatment.

By the time I attended the Kushi seminar, I had read enough proponent literature to shortcircuit my infatuation with macrobiotics. Nonetheless, I received a long overdue intellectual "cold shower," for I found there not an alternate or complementary system of healthcare but an antiscientific patchwork of a cult.

Yoga, ayurveda, and macrobiotics are distinctly Eastern philosophies. The next chapter deals with an American aberration—the Edgar Cayce tradition.

7

The Edgar Cayce Tradition

Edgar Cayce (1877–1945) was a precursor of New Age trance channeling. Biographer Jess Stern dubbed him the "sleeping prophet." A poorly educated photographer and Sunday-school teacher with no medical training whatsoever, Cayce gained nationwide renown for "diagnosing" illnesses and prescribing "remedies" while in a self-induced trance. Between 1910 and his death, he gave well over fourteen thousand "psychic readings." His current promoters claim:

> He could see into the future and the past ... describe present far-off events as they were happening; and ... astound doctors with his x-ray vision of the human body. His readings—his words while in this state—were carefully transcribed while they were spoken. He is undoubtedly the most documented psychic who ever lived. And the accuracy of his predictions has been put at well over ninety percent! At his death, he left a legacy of thousands of case histories that science is still at a loss to explain completely.

"To the Will of God"

Cayce was born and raised on a tobacco farm near Hopkinsville, Kentucky, in the small, isolated, rural community of Christian County. In *Edgar Cayce on Diet and Health* (1969), his son, Hugh Lynn Cayce (1907–1982), wrote: "At the age of six or seven, he told his parents that he was able to see and talk to 'visions,' sometimes of relatives who had recently died. His parents attributed this to the overactive imagination of a lonely child who had been influenced by the dramatic language of the revival meetings which were popular in that section of the country." *Edgar Cayce Speaks* (1969) states that as a child Cayce was "troubled" and rather "backward," constantly seeking solace and refuge in the Bible under the influence of his devoutly religious mother. He quit school after completing the seventh grade.

Cayce's career as a clairvoyant began in 1901 after a session with an amateur hypnotist, Al C. Layne. Layne had become an osteopath by means of a correspondence course. In a trance, Cayce supposedly diagnosed the source of his own persistent laryngitis and prescribed a cure for it. In *There Is a River: The Story of Edgar Cayce* (1945), Thomas Sugrue stated that during "self-hypnosis," Cayce told Layne "in a clear, unafflicted voice":

> In the normal state, this body is unable to speak, due to a partial paralysis of the inferior muscles of the vocal cords, produced by nerve strain. This is a psychological condition producing a physical effect. This may be removed by increasing the circulation to the affected parts by suggestion while in this unconscious condition.

Layne proposed that they use this method to cure others and asked Cayce to diagnose and prescribe for a stomach ailment Layne had had for years. On the following afternoon, Cayce entered a trance and prescribed patent medicines, simple mixtures, a diet, and a set of exercises. Layne responded: "If it works, our fortunes are made!" Within three weeks, Layne's condition improved considerably and he announced his intention to practice "suggestive therapeutics" and osteopathy. He opened his office months later with Cayce as his "silent partner." According to *Mysteries of Mind, Space & Time—The Unexplained* (1992), whenever Cayce decided to quit giving "readings," he lost his voice or developed a severe headache. As news of the "healings" spread, thousands sought his help. In *The Outer Limits of Edgar Cayce's Power* (1971), Cayce's sons stated that the transcripts of the readings comprise over fifty thousand single-spaced typewritten pages and more than ten million words.

Cayce offered guidance both to persons in attendance and to distant correspondents; he supposedly needed only the individual's name and address. In *A Seer Out of Season: The Life of Edgar Cayce* (1989), Jungian psychotherapist Harmon Hartzell Bro, Ph.D., states that the crux of Cayce's trance-counseling was "disciplined emptying [of the self] which would enable one's habitual will to conform more closely to the will of God, and one's mind to be transformed by the renewing action of larger Reality." Allegedly drawing upon the "akashic records"—which he described as "records written on time and space"—Cayce revealed "facts" about mythical civilizations, astrological influences, "past lives," and future events. However, Time-Life Books' *Psychic Powers* describes two instances in which he prescribed for patients who had already died.

In middle age, Cayce began regularly accepting payment for his readings. In them, he described vitamins as "creative forces" that work with "body energies" and from which glands take "those necessary influences to supply the energies to enable the various organs of the body to reproduce themselves." He stated that the top portion of carrots contains "vital energies which stimulate the optic reactions between the kidneys and the optics." "The Creator's forces are in every force," he said. "There is healing in the power and might of the love of God." He also stated: "All healing forces are within, not without! The applications from without are merely to create within a coordinating mental and spiritual force." Cayce declared that it was "well for everyone to make a study of astrology."

A motif of Cayce advocates stems from a leading question in the readings: "Should the Christ Consciousness be described as the awareness within each soul, imprinted in pattern on the mind and waiting to be awakened by the will, of the soul's oneness with God?" Cayce replied: "Correct. That's the idea exactly!" He likened the supposed interrelationship of body, mind, and spirit to that of Father, Son, and Holy Spirit—the components of the Christian god.

Cayce's Legacies

Several organizations have grown up around Cayce's work. The headquarters of the Association for Research and Enlightenment (A.R.E.), which occupies an entire city block in Virginia Beach, is home to four of them: Atlantic University, the Harold J. Reilly School of Massotherapy, the Edgar Cayce Foundation, and A.R.E., Inc.

According to its 1989–90 catalog, Atlantic University opened with a traditional undergraduate program in 1931 and operated for about a year and a half before closing. The university's 1993–94 catalog states that it reopened in 1985 as a graduate school. Although it is not accredited, it awards a master of arts degree in "transpersonal studies." The catalog's "purpose statement" defines this as "an interdisciplinary field which includes psychology, philosophy, sociology, history, literature, religion, and science." The catalog explains:

> The founding principle of transpersonal studies is the existence of a dimension to human nature greater than the individual. The transpersonal thesis is that connecting with this larger part of oneself is instrumental to creativity, health, and full human performance.

Courses cover astrology, dreamwork, *I Ching*, Jungian psychology, palmistry, psychometry, tarot, transpersonal counseling, and processes to "balance and transform" human "energies." Students may pursue the master's degree largely through home study. The November/December 1993 issue of *Venture Inward*, the magazine of the A.R.E. and the Edgar Cayce Foundation, announced the school's plan to offer a "comprehensive curriculum in holistic health and holistic living," including "masters level courses, certificate courses for healthcare practitioners, and a self-care course for laypersons." Atlantic's January–October 1993 progress report stated that the school had increased the number of correspondence courses applicable to its "master's degree" from four to eight, had instituted a second option whereby graduate students may bypass writing a thesis, and had applied for accreditation to the National Home Study Council. According to the January/February 1994 issue of *Venture Inward*, the "Holistic Health and Holistic Living" curriculum covers "the body, mind, and spirit model of the multi-dimensional human being" and "the concept of energy."

The Reilly School, which operates under the auspices of the university, opened in 1931, closed within a year and a half, and reopened in 1986. It is the namesake of a physical therapist, reputedly with eight degrees, to whom Cayce made hundreds of explicit references in the readings. For example, during one reading, Cayce advised:

> Talk to Dr. Reilly about it. He has had experiences with thousands of cases. [He] is the one that does just as the information suggests that gets real results, whether it appears to be in accord with what other people have told them or not.

Harold J. Reilly was born in New York City in 1895. He graduated from the American School of Naturopathy and the American School of Chiropractic, both founded by Benedict Lust (see Chapter 8). For several years, Reilly studied at the Kellogg Institute in Battle Creek, Michigan, under Seventh-day Adventist Dr. John Harvey Kellogg, the inventor of prepackaged breakfast cereals and author of *Rational Hydrotherapy* (1900). In 1935, Reilly opened the fashionable Reilly Health Institute at New York's Rockefeller Center. He closed the institute in 1965, donated his physiotherapy equipment to the A.R.E., and directed the Edgar Cayce Foundation's physiotherapy and rehabilitation clinic in Virginia Beach for at least ten years. One of Reilly's books, *The Edgar Cayce Handbook for Health Through Drugless Therapy* (1975), cites Cayce's advice to a businessman during a reading:

> There is nothing better ... [than peanut-oil massages]. They do supply energies to the body. And, just as indicated in other suggestions—those

who would eat 2 to 3 almonds each day need never fear cancer. Those who would take a peanut oil rub each week need never fear arthritis.

Certified by the Commonwealth of Virginia, the Reilly School offers a 600-hour diploma program in massage therapy. The program includes instruction in diet, foot reflexology, hydrotherapy, and preventive healthcare based on the Cayce readings. The school has also offered workshops on biofeedback, Cayce home remedies, and iridology.

The Edgar Cayce Foundation, chartered in 1948, was formed to preserve the Cayce readings and documentation.

The A.R.E., cofounded by Hugh Lynn Cayce in 1931, functions as an eclectic New Age nerve center, from which emanates a steady flow of seminars and publications. A 1991 brochure describes it as "a living network of people who are finding a deeper meaning in life through the psychic work of Edgar Cayce." In 1976, Hugh Lynn became board chairman and his son, Charles Thomas Cayce, became president. A.R.E. headquarters, a modern three-story building in Virginia Beach, includes a visitor/conference center, a library, and the A.R.E. bookstore. It receives more than forty thousand visitors and conference attendees annually. With more than fifty thousand volumes, the library has one of the world's largest collections of parapsychological and metaphysical literature.

Standard A.R.E. membership costs $30 per year, but nine-month "introductory" memberships are available for $15 or $20. Members receive the bimonthly *Venture Inward* and can borrow books from the A.R.E. Library, join a study group, and attend or send their children to the A.R.E.'s summer camp in the Appalachian foothills. They also may obtain referrals to over four hundred practitioners who use the Cayce approach. A November 1993 mailing stated that A.R.E. had about thirty thousand members and that there are Edgar Cayce Centers in Costa Rica, Ecuador, England, Japan, and Sweden.

The A.R.E. invites members to participate in "home research projects" in which they perform activities pertaining to such matters as astrology, numerology, and synchronicity and report the results. Participation is free for some "self-study" projects, but others cost from $17 to about $30 per person. A 1991 issue of the *Home Research Project* bulletin states: "The main commitment of A.R.E. as a research organization is to encourage you to test concepts in the Cayce readings and to look for—and expect—results." Study groups center on such concerns as diet, the laws of reincarnation (karma), metaphysical dream interpretation, and the spiritual legacies of ancient Egypt and Atlantis. According to an A.R.E. letter, "Thousands gather together in small groups all over the country to study and apply spiritual principles in daily living." A.R.E. mailings to prospective members state: "There is no human problem for which the Cayce predictions do not offer hope." A.R.E. "research reports," based on the Cayce readings, are available on a wide variety of topics, including scar removal, warts, arthritis, diabetes, and multiple sclerosis.

Each year, the A.R.E. holds dozens of conferences in Virginia Beach and various other cities. They have covered such subjects as angels, astrology ("the key to self-discovery"), Atlantean science and technology, Bach flower therapy, chakra healing, homeopathy, "intuitive healing," reincarnation, UFOs, weight control, and "holistic" financial management. A flyer for a 1992 "psychic training" seminar states: "You are already psychic.... You only need to become aware of it!"

The A.R.E. Bookstore, which sells direct and by mail, features many books about Cayce, including *The Complete Edgar Cayce Readings* on CD-ROM, priced at $500. It also carries a large selection of uncritical books and videotapes on supernaturalistic topics, including bioenergy, chakras, the "human energy field," crystal healing, the "healing power" of prayer, guardian angels, Japanese astrology ("nine star ki"), "magic" flower remedies, "money magnetism," reincarnation, and the souls of animals.

The A.R.E. Clinic

Another item sold by the bookstore is the *Physician's Reference Notebook* by William A. McGarey, M.D., and associates. McGarey is board chairperson and a cofounder of the A.R.E. Clinic in Phoenix, Arizona. The book offers treatment recommendations based on the Cayce readings for over fifty diseases and conditions, including baldness, breast cancer, color blindness, diabetes, hemophilia, hydrocephalus, leukemia, multiple sclerosis, muscular dystrophy, stroke, stuttering, and syphilis. According to the *Notebook*: (1) baldness is most often caused by glandular insufficiency and spinal lesions (subluxations); (2) color blindness is caused by the conduct of the afflicted person in a past life, and treatment should include spinal adjustments and a diet consisting mostly of alkali-producing foods; (3) hemophilia is correctable, "a simple case of a deep-seated defect in the assimilations of the body," and treatment of newborns so afflicted should consist primarily of the addition of blood pudding to the diet; (4) obesity is caused principally by an excess of starches in the diet, and treatment should include the elimination of most starches; and (5) psoriasis is caused by a thinning of the intestinal walls, which "allows toxic products from the intestinal tract to leak into the circulatory system and find their way into the lymph flow of the skin."

In an interview in *Health Talks* (1989), McGarey stated: "The philosophy behind the A.R.E. clinic is that everyone is a whole human being. . . . created in the image of God." He lamented: "When doctors fail to recognize the spiritual aspect of the human being, they miss the most important part." "Our destiny is getting back to our spiritual origin," he said. "Then there is a different kind of emphasis on healing; you do not get tied up with modalities. Healing is more of a spiritual event. The cells within the body go through a change when the individual . . . realizes that Divine source of his life."

McGarey's methods include acuscope therapy, biofeedback, dream analysis, and the laying on of hands. In *Health Talks*, McGarey said that acuscope therapy involves "normalization of the acupressure points within the body." An A.R.E. Clinic flyer describes the acuscope as "a computerized, flexible system for applying just the proper amount of micro-current to the appropriate areas of the body and obtaining accurate feedback about the results of the application." It claims that the acuscope "helps to balance the electrical current of the body which is necessary for healing." Acuscope therapy is allegedly "a practical, effective application of Energy Medicine, the medicine of the future."

In the July/August 1993 issue of *Venture Inward*, former A.R.E. trustee Rudy Barden states that after undergoing surgery for bladder cancer in December 1992, he refused chemotherapy and instead attended the clinic's eleven-day residential Temple Beautiful Program. He writes:

> The treatments . . . included exercise, meditation, visualization, dietary changes, colonics [enemas], massage, castor oil packs, beef extract, carbon ash, ultraviolet light, energy medicine, dream interpretation, biofeedback, spinal manipulations, lectures, and counseling. Ridding the body of toxins and poisons, building up the immune system, and helping each of us to determine why we got cancer, what it was supposed to accomplish, and what caused it, were very important. I got my answers.

The clinic markets more than one hundred fifty products to the general public through a department called the Cayce Corner. The products include herbal teas and "tonics," homeopathic "remedies," cosmetics and shampoos, electrical devices, books, and videocassettes. The "Radio-Active Appliance" and the "Radiac Impedance Device," for example, purportedly meet Cayce's specifications. A catalog equates the two devices and states:

> Who can benefit from the device? Cayce said, "Everyone!" The device is so easy to use: just place it in a bucket of ice, attach the electrodes to your wrist and ankle with Velcro, and relax. You can even use it while you sleep at night!

What does it do? According to the readings, it draws your auric energy in through the red electrode, filters and refines it, then sends it back into your body through the black electrode. In this way it balances your mental, emotional, and physical energies. Cayce said the harmonization with the Creative Forces becomes so great that the days you use it will be "lucky" days!

According to the January/February 1994 issue of *Venture Inward*, McGarey relinquished his medical license in November 1993 under pressure from the Arizona State Board of Medical Examiners. The article states that the board had investigated the A.R.E. Clinic in 1991 and subsequently censured McGarey for "inappropriate therapy" and directed him to take the state medical licensing exam. McGarey failed the exam twice and, according to the article, concluded that it was "an unfair test of his competence as a physician." In the same issue, McGarey, then 74 years old, stated:

I would like to establish a College of Holistic Healing here at the Clinic, a place where lay people could learn how to take care of themselves, their families, and friends. Simple ideas, simple truths. Simple steps that might just help us grow closer to the Divine and thus fulfill more completely our soul purpose for being here in the earth plane in the first place.

The Bottom Line

"Spiritual healing" posits and emphasizes a "bright side" to illness and thus often provides comfort in the form of unrealistic hope. The "spiritual healer" who focuses this hope on "cleansing," "spiritual reclamation," and "life after death" may claim that healing occurred even if the patient died from the "blessed" and "transformative" illness. Deathbed sentimentality and claims of postmortem effects beneficial to the patient are outrageous "consolation prizes." Like other forms of "spiritual healing," the Edgar Cayce approach traffics in the hope of everlasting life and the fear of personal nonexistence, feeding into and feeding on a climate of "pro-paranormal" credulity.

Part III

Pseudonatural "Healing"

8

Back to "Supernature"

In "alternative" healthcare, the word "nature" often denotes a salutary, creative, guiding force—the "vital force," the "Universal Mother," or God. Unncessary capitalization of the word *nature* usually signifies theism or supernaturalistic pantheism.

According to pantheism, the terms "God" and "nature" are synonymous. In its supernaturalistic form, pantheism ascribes supernatural phenomena or a morality to "nature." Bob Bloomfield, former executive officer for Britain's International Federation of Practitioners of Natural Therapeutics, implied supernaturalistic pantheism in *The Mystique of Healing* (1985):

> There can be, surely, only one true source of healing energy and that is nature itself; but we all have our philosophies, our religions, our beliefs or lack of them. There are many terms applied to the ultimate source of healing. . . . God, Mother Nature, the Cosmic Source, the Life Force, Christ Light. Call it what you will—it is there! It does not really matter what your religious, philosophical or semantic approach to the question might be.
>
> There are a number of ways of drawing upon that single, secret source of healing energy.

"Natural Laws"

Scientists define natural laws as *descriptions* (explanations) of relationships between objects, events, and forces, based on meticulous observation and precise reasoning. The law of gravity is a well-known example. Such relationships are not inherently directive and do not ordain human behaviors. Advocates of "alternative" healthcare, however, use the term "natural laws" to connote a morality of nature, and many theists hold that the word "law" implies the existence of a lawgiver (God). In *Health at the Crossroads: Exploring the Conflict Between Natural Healing and Conventional Medicine* (1988), Dean Black, Ph.D., former president of two health-food companies, writes:

> There is some higher principle that must first be honored. . . . *Nature has its own laws and may not allow intrusion without revenge.* . . . Our only choice is to seek a way of getting along with nature that doesn't pit us against her, that instead allies us with her, capturing her strength for our own.

In *Fit for Life II: Living Health* (1988), Harvey Diamond, a proponent of Natural Hygiene (see next chapter), states in boldface:

> **THE TRUE CAUSE OF IMPAIRED HEALTH LIES IN OUR FAILURE TO COMPLY WITH THE LAWS AND REQUIREMENTS OF LIFE. ALL HEALTH PROBLEMS ARISE FROM THE ABUSE OF NATURAL LAWS. . . . LIVING HEALTHFULLY IS NOT AN ART THAT WE MUST LEARN, IT IS AN INSTINCTIVE WAY OF LIFE TO WHICH WE MUST RETURN!**

In the same book, Harvey's wife Marilyn states that "nerve energy" is the body's "most important commodity." However, she says: "Nobody really understands its essential nature, but nobody knows exactly what electricity is either and we use it just the same." Later she declares: "Our breath *is* us; *it is our life force.*"

In a Fall 1993 mailing titled *Tomorrow's Health*, "complementary physician" Robert C. Atkins, M.D., warned:

> Don't try to play tricks on Mother Nature. . . . You'll soon find that she has her own tricks, and if you keep annoying her, she'll get even with you!
> Stay on her side. Stick to natural, nutritional remedies when you can: They're *enabling* agents. Avoid drugs when you can: They're *blocking* agents.

Such writers do not refer to the nature (material world) examined by physicists and scientific philosophers, but to the prescriptive "Nature" of theologians, who hold that the material world is the work of God.

Black describes "natural healing":

> The very gentleness that pleases patients and tends to avoid side effects also produces a certain conceptual and practical fuzziness that makes

proving that natural healing [is effective] almost impossible, at least to the satisfaction of classically trained scientists. . . .

The [alternative] logic of natural healing . . . leaves an opening for charlatans. Unlike [scientific] medicine, it places little value on explaining how a therapy works, so it doesn't concern itself with theory. Intending not to meddle, natural healing hardly ever considers what actually goes on inside the body. As a result, it doesn't depend nearly so much as medicine on having scientifically trained practitioners. In fact, much of natural healing is scarcely more complex than common sense. . . .

And natural healing is much more diverse than medicine. Anything that can affect the body's adaptive powers—which is virtually everything—may become part of natural healing. . . . Natural healing . . . tends to be much more loosely defined than medicine, and hardly concise enough to allow such things as discipline-wide licensing boards of the sort that govern medicine. . . .

So charlatans who choose health as their scam are much more likely to venture into natural healing than medicine.

"Natural healing" includes such supernaturalistic methods and systems as absent healing, acupuncture and acupressure, aikido, the Alexander technique, anthroposophy, applied kinesiology, astrology, ayurveda, bioenergetics, the Edgar Cayce approach, the charismatic movement, fundamentalist chiropractic, Christian Science, cranial osteopathy, dianetics, exorcism, hydropathy and kneipping, iridology, *jin shin jitsu* and *jin shin do*, Jungian psychology, the laying on of hands, lomi-lomi, macrobiotics, mesmerism, nature cure, naturopathy, orgonomy, past-life therapy, polarity therapy, primal therapy, psychic healing, radiesthesia and radionics, reflexology, reiki, rolfing, shamanism, tai chi, therapeutic touch, Touch for Health, transcendental meditation, yoga, and "vibrational medicine" ("vibrational healing"). "Vibrational medicine" includes aromatherapy, chakra therapy, color therapy, crystal therapy, flower essence therapy, gem therapy, homeopathy, psychic surgery, and toning (a form of music therapy). In *Natural Medicine* (1980), British journalist Brian Inglis wrote:

Natural medicine has always thrown out offshoots. Some keep in the public eye; some are preserved only by tiny groups of devotees; some disappear. Dissatisfaction with orthodox medicine, as well as improving the prospects for the established ["alternative"] therapies, has led to the revival of others which had seemed moribund. Some of them will fade away again; but if natural medicine is going to be brought into [mainstream] health services, it will need to accumulate any of them which expand.

The Striving for "Purity"

Modern "natural healing" is traceable to Vincenz Priessnitz (1791–1851) of Silesia and the appearance of hydropathy, or "water cure." "Hydropathy" refers to the internal and external use of water as a near-panacea. In *Alternative Medicine and American Religious Life* (1989), Prof. Robert C. Fuller writes: "The theoretical rationale of hydropathy centered upon the power of water to restore humans to a condition of purity."

As a shepherd, Priessnitz reportedly often observed injured animals go to streams, immerse their limbs, and emerge in much better conditions. He thus became convinced that pure cold water was a therapeutic marvel. He tested his conviction on villagers with strains, bruises, and broken limbs. Deeming the treatment successful, Priessnitz applied it to other ailments, always using water not warmer than 88°F. He established spas where patients who were either seriously ill or chronically disabled took an ice-cold "torrent shower bath" outdoors for two to five minutes, then an "air-and-water" bath. His "dripping sheet treatment" involved the wringing out of a linen sheet in cold water, its placement over the shoulders of the patient, and subsequent vigorous massage. Practitioners applied this treatment to cholera and to diseases of the brain, heart, kidneys, liver, and lungs.

In the United States, hydropathy's two eminent spokespersons were Joel Shew and Russell Thacker Trall, M.D. (1812–1877), who together opened a hydropathic institution in Lebanon Springs, New York, in 1845. Shew developed a "comprehensive" hydropathic regimen involving fresh air, diet, sleep, and clothing. He claimed his system could remedy cholera, constipation, fever, hiccups, poisoning, gastric bleeding, and digestive problems. Other hydropaths added to this roster: bladder infections, diseases of the ear, gout, malaria, obesity, whooping cough, and excessive sexual desire.

The hydropathy movement peaked around 1850 and almost disappeared after Trall's death. However, Sebastian Kneipp (1821–1897), a Bavarian Catholic priest, revived it later in the century. Kneipp had supposedly cured himself of tuberculosis with hydropathy. He combined it with herbalism and lifestyle. In *So sollt ihr leben*—translated as "Thus Thou Shalt Live"—he advocated a return to "Nature." Kneipp recommended wearing coarse home-made underpants, spending most of each day outdoors, walking barefoot on wet (dewy) grass, and running on snow.

Edward Wicksted Lane, M.D., developed the idea of "hygienic medicine" in Britain. In *Hydropathy: or Hygienic Medicine* (1859), he stated that the term "hydropathy" covered only one aspect of hygienic medicine; that nature was "constantly endeavoring to work out her own cure"; and that hygienic medicine relied on air, diet, exercise, water, and "healthy mental and moral influences."

Hydropathy thus became the hub of nature cure—a "natural" lifestyle upon which accumulated a medley of "treatments" known collectively as naturopathy.

In a 1985 issue of *Culture, Medicine and Psychiatry*, Thomas W. Maretzki and Edward Seidler wrote:

> Natural healing is based on traditional ideas about vitalistic forces and defense mechanisms involved in the body processes of health mainte-nance and healing, and the role of outside stimuli . . . acting on these processes either beneficially or as irritants. Among these are water, air, hot and cold, sun and altitude, the ocean, minerals as contained in water, naturally grown foods and medicinal herbs. . . .
>
> Naturopathy as experiential medicine . . . does not rely on controlled experiments. It combines knowledge preserved in tradition with familiarity gained through careful clinical observation of the patient to establish the progression and waning of an illness.

Naturopathy

Naturopathy—so-called natural therapeutics or natural medicine— is a com-posite "healing" tradition touted as "drugless" and reliant solely upon "natural" powers. Naturopathy did not spring from a unified doctrine and lacks coherence in both theory and practice. It is characterized by a miscellany of vitalistic approaches, which include acupuncture (including ear acupuncture and electroacupuncture), Chinese herbalism, homeopathy (described below), *jin shin* (a form of acupressure), Jungian psychotherapy, moxibustion and cup-ping, ortho-bionomy, *tui na*, and zone therapy (reflexology). However, naturo-paths generally agree that a "life force" or "vital curative force"—misrepre-sented as the Hippocratic *vis medicatrix naturae*—normally flows through the body in various channels, and that blockages cause "imbalances" leading to disease. Literature from Bastyr University states:

> Naturopathic physicians seek to restore and maintain optimum health in their patients by emphasizing nature's inherent capacity to heal, the vis medicatrix naturae. . . . Naturopathic medicine recognizes an inherent ability in the body which is ordered and intelligent. Naturo-pathic physicians act to identify and remove obstacles to recovery, and to facilitate and augment this healing ability.

Naturopaths claim to remove or treat the underlying causes of disease on physical, mental/emotional, spiritual, social, and other levels. They further claim to facilitate the response of the "life force" to illness through "cleansing" and "detoxification." They deem anything that supposedly dampens the "life force" an underlying cause. The American Association of Naturopathic Physicians (AANP) states: "Naturopathic medicine has its own unique body of knowledge, evolved and refined for centuries." In a 1991 article, naturopath Robert H. Sorge—founder of the Abunda Life Health Hotel in Asbury Park, New Jersey—states that the major contributors to an elevated cholesterol level include "devitalized foods," worry, fear, anxiety, autointoxication, "metabolic imbalance," "colon toxicity," malabsorption, and "liver sluggishness." Sorge's "N.D." degree came from an unaccredited correspondence school that promoted spondylotherapy—a system of pseudodiagnosis and pseudotherapy that involved percussing the spine. (Albert Abrams, the originator of radionics, pioneered spondylotherapy, publishing books on the subject in 1909 and 1910.)

Most naturopaths believe that virtually all diseases are within their scope of practice. They offer treatment at their offices and at spas where patients may stay for several weeks. Along with the vitalistic approaches listed above, their methods include: biofeedback, hypnotherapy, fasting, Natural Hygiene, nutritional supplementation, exercise, enemas and other forms of hydrotherapy, diathermy (heat treatment), ultrasound, spinal manipulation, "natural childbirth care," and minor surgery. Naturopaths are legally permitted to use x-rays for diagnosis but not for treatment. The most comprehensive naturopathic publications, *A Textbook of Natural Medicine* (for students and professionals) and the *Encyclopedia of Natural Medicine* (for laypersons), recommend dietary measures, vitamins, minerals, and/or herbs for more than seventy health problems, ranging from acne to AIDS.

Dr. John H. Scheel, a German-born homeopath who practiced in New York City, coined the word "naturopathy" in 1895 to describe his methods of healthcare. In 1902, he sold the rights to the name to Benedict Lust, a disciple of Father Kneipp who had come to the United States in 1892 to promote hydropathy. Lust was largely responsible for naturopathy's growth in this country. He acquired degrees in chiropractic, homeopathy, naturopathy, and osteopathy, and a medical license based on his homeopathy degree. In the United States, the heyday of naturopathy occurred during the 1920s and 1930s. Its popularity waned over the next three decades as scientific medicine developed and chiropractic schools stopped granting naturopathy diplomas.

Bodybuilder Bernarr Macfadden (1868–1955), another naturopathic luminary, was a supporter of homeopathy, chiropractic, and autology—a pseudoscientific system based on the notion that moderation, equality, work, and love are sufficient to treat disease. He founded the Bernarr Macfadden Institute of Physical Culture in New York in 1905, which became two schools in 1913: the American College of Physical Education and the Macfadden College of Physcultopathy. In 1915, the latter school became the International College of Drugless Physicians. "Physcultopathy" refers to the "curative" phase of Macfadden's philosophy of "physical culture." Physical culture promoted exercise, fasting, hydrotherapy, nudism, "natural" foods, and abstention from alcohol, coffee, tea, most drugs, and tobacco. Macfadden also introduced Cosmotarianism, a religion whose paramount doctrine was that the sure way to heaven lay in cherishing one's own body. In *Barefoot In Eden: The Macfadden Plan for Health, Charm, and Long-lasting Youth* (1962), Macfadden's fourth wife, Johnnie Lee Macfadden, wrote:

> Macfadden was not a vegetarian, as so many people believed. He experimented with a vegetarian diet for a time, but decided that the body needed the tissue-building elements of meat protein for top energy. In his own case, he felt that meat increased his virility, and he always prescribed it for his patients.

In *Fads and Quackery in Healing* (1932), Morris Fishbein, M.D., editor of the *Journal of the American Medical Association* and an influential opponent of quackery, wrote:

> Naturopathy and the allied cults represent capitalization for purposes of financial gain of the old advice that outdoor life, good diet, enough exercise, and rest are conducive to health and longevity. When these simple principles can be linked with the printing of worthless pamphlets, intricate apparatus, or faith cures, the formulas yield gold. . . .
> The real naturopaths . . . advocated natural living and healed by the use of sunlight, baths, fresh air, and cold water, but there is little money to be made by these methods. Hence the modern naturopath embraces every form of healing that offers opportunity for exploitation . . . . from aeropathy [wherein "the patient is baked in a hot oven"] to zonotherapy [reflexology].

In 1968, the U.S. Department of Health, Education, and Welfare (HEW) recommended against coverage of naturopathy under Medicare. HEW's report concluded:

> Naturopathic theory and practice are not based upon the body of basic knowledge related to health, disease, and health care which has been widely accepted by the scientific community. Moreover, irrespective of its theory, the scope and quality of naturopathic education do not prepare the practitioner to make an adequate diagnosis and provide appropriate treatment.

The doctor of naturopathy (N.D.) degree is now available from three full-time schools of naturopathy and a few correspondence schools. The curriculum at the full-time institutions includes two years of basic science courses such as human anatomy and physiology and two years of clinical naturopathy. In 1987, the U.S. Secretary of Education approved the Council on Naturopathic Medical Education (CNME) as an accrediting agency. Unfortunately, accreditation is not based on the soundness of what is taught, but on such factors as record-keeping, physical assets, financial status, makeup of the governing body, catalog characteristics, nondiscrimination policy, and self-evaluation system.

The leading naturopathy school, Bastyr University, in Seattle, Washington, is accredited by the CNME. Besides its N.D. program, Bastyr offers a B.S. degree program in Natural Health Sciences with majors in nutrition and Oriental medicine, and M.S. programs in nutrition and acupuncture. Bastyr also provides health-food retailers and their employees with home-study programs that promote "natural" approaches for the gamut of disease. The other four-year schools are the National College of Naturopathic Medicine in Portland, Oregon, and the recently opened Southwest College of Naturopathic Medicine and Health Sciences in Scottsdale, Arizona. Most of the latter's initial funding came from companies that market dietary supplements, homeopathic products, and/or herbal remedies.

Naturopathic licensing laws exist in only seven states and the District of Columbia. Several other states have laws that permit naturopaths to practice, but most states do not officially allow them to do so. A directory in the January/February 1992 issue of *East West Natural Health* lists nearly four hundred naturopaths with practices in twenty-seven states, the District of Columbia, and Puerto Rico. The total number of practitioners is unknown, but includes chiropractors and acupuncturists who practice naturopathy. Medicare and most health insurance policies do not cover naturopathic services. In 1993, an AANP official said that his group represented more than eight hundred naturopaths and that licensure efforts were underway in sixteen states.

Homeopathy

Homeopathy, a form of "energy medicine" developed by German physician Samuel Hahnemann (1755–1843), is perhaps the preeminent naturopathic subsystem. In the April 1993 issue of *Let's Live*, homeopathic pharmacist John A. Borneman III wrote:

The naturopaths are leading the way toward training physicians in homeopathy. . . . Naturopathic physicians have taken an active role in the traditional homeopathic community. The major naturopathic organizations are strongly oriented toward homeopathy. . . . Naturopathic physicians have been well represented at the National Center for Homeopathy's annual meetings, where their presentations have been enthusiastically received.

The March 1985 issue of *FDA Consumer* stated: "As Americans have become increasingly infatuated in the past few years with all things 'natural,' homeopathy has also had a resurgence as a result of this back-to-nature movement, offering a 'non-chemical' way of treating illness without side effects." Homeopathy is still going strong.

Is homeopathy natural? Proponents say it is. For example, one mamufacturer of "supplements" Nature's Way Products, Inc., calls its line of homeopathic "remedies" Medicine From Nature™. Another, Natra-Bio, describes homeopathic "remedies" as natural medicines that do not have side effects. Its homeopathic reference manual states: "In homeopathic medicine, the body's natural capacity to heal itself is safely and effectively enhanced." Homeopathic Educational Services in Berkeley, California, calls homeopathy "a natural pharmaceutical science."

Actually, homeopathy's theoretical basis is supernaturalistic. In *Homoeopathic Medicine* (1975), proponent Harris L. Coulter, Ph.D., wrote:

> From Hahnemann onwards, the homeopathic physicians have characterized the processes of health and disease in vitalistic terms. They have talked of a "vital force," "power of recovery," or "natural force" in the body—a force which reacts to external stimuli. . . .
>
> The vitalistic assumption is of primordial importance for homeopathic therapeutics, since it imposes a particular interpretation of the symptom. Regardless of how disagreeable or even painful it may be, the symptom is still the visible manifestation of the organism's reactive power. And since this reactive power always strives for cure . . . and always strives to adjust the balance between the body and its environment, the symptoms are not the signs of a morbific [pathological], but of a curative, process. They point out to the physician the route taken by the body in coping with some particular stress; hence they are the best guides to treatment. Since the body's reactive force endeavors to cope with a given stress by producing *a particular set of symptoms*, the physician's duty is to promote the development of this very set of symptoms.

Below I briefly describe six of the major homeopathic theories, all of which originated with Hahnemann.

• *The law of similars ("like cures like"):* According to this "law," the most effective remedy for a particular disease is that which can produce in a healthy person all the symptoms of the disease with administration of a significant amount. For example, to eliminate nausea, a homeopath might prescribe a preparation containing a minuscule amount of ipecac, a drug that in therapeutic amounts induces nausea.

• *The doctrine of individualization (the rule of the single remedy):* Some homeopaths prescribe only one "remedy" at a time. In selecting it, they apparently consider not only the symptoms that prompted the patient's visit but variables such as mood, food preferences, and reactions to weather. Seemingly, the ideal homeopathic "remedy" is that which in pharmacologic amounts would cause in a healthy person all the symptoms, moods, preferences, and idiosyncrasies reported by the patient.

• *The doctrine of the minimum dose ("less is more"):* Homeopaths maintain that the intake of minuscule—or even nonexistent—"doses" of peculiarly selected substances triggers healing without side effects.

• *The doctrine of potentization ("dynamization"):* Homeopaths claim that the succussion (shaking) and progressive dilution of a "therapeutic" substance during the preparation of a "remedy" increase the effectiveness of the "remedy" and remove the toxicity of the substance. Purportedly, manufacturers of homeopathic products repeatedly dilute soluble substances with alcohol or water and shake the solution; similarly, they repeatedly crush insoluble substances and thin them with lactose. A pamphlet for consumers published by Standard Homeopathic Co., in Los Angeles, California, defines "vital force" as a "natural defense reaction" and states: "Homeopathic 'high' potencies . . . contain only the most minute amount of the basic remedy; but the remedy has been 'potentized' by vigorous shaking at each step of reduction or dilution in order to enhance the remedy's therapeutic effectiveness." The pamphlet further states that, generally, "lower potencies"—i.e., preparations containing relatively large amounts of the "basic remedy"—are "appropriate and effectively used by the consumer," and that "high potencies"—i.e., preparations containing little or none of the "basic remedy"—are "the province of the trained Homeopathic prescriber."

• *The theory of the chronic miasms:* Hahnemann coined the term "miasms" to refer to the three hereditary sources he posited for all chronic diseases resistant to homeopathic treatment. He labeled these alleged propensities "sycotic" (gonorrheal), syphilitic, and "psoric." "Psora," the original miasm, supposedly manifests itself as skin diseases such as scabies. It is analogous to the Christian idea of original sin—an alleged hereditary predisposition to evil. Some homeopaths reject the miasmic (or miasmatic) theory, while others adopt it uncritically and interpret it metaphorically.

• *The doctrine of the vital force:* Hahnemann coined the word "dynamis" to refer to the "vital force." His final theory held that the "vital force" is the source of all biological phenomena, that it becomes deranged during illness, and that appropriate homeopathic "remedies" work by restoring the "vital force." In *Homeopathy: Medicine of the New Man* (1987), teacher and practitioner George Vithoulkas stated that one proof of the existence of the "vital force" is "the fact that when the disturbed organism of a patient is properly tuned through the administration of the right homeopathic remedy, the patient not only experiences the alleviation of symptoms, but also has the feeling that life once again is harmoniously flowing through him."

All of these theories clash with modern scientific knowledge.

The Bottom Line

"Natural healing" is a tangle of vitalism, spiritism, theism, supernaturalistic pantheism, and mysticism. Proponents use the word "natural" to suggest that the theories underlying their systems are consistent with "natural laws." These "laws," however, are nothing more than traditional beliefs. I call supernaturalistic methods that purport to be natural *pseudonatural* because they falsely imply that scientific methods violate the laws of nature.

The following chapter deals with Natural Hygiene, an austere form of naturopathy.

9

Natural Hygiene

Natural Hygiene, a Spartan form of naturopathy, is a comprehensive philosophy of health and "natural living" whose ideal diet consists exclusively of vegetables, fruits, nuts, and seeds—all uncooked and minimally processed. Natural Hygiene recommends fasting, whether one is sick or healthy, and denounces virtually all medical treatments—including herbal remedies and nutritional supplements. *Health Science,* the official membership journal of the American Natural Hygiene Society, summarizes Hygienic philosophy on its masthead:

> Health is the result of natural living. When people live in harmony with their physiological needs, health is the inevitable result. By supplying the organism with its basic requirements (natural, unadulterated food; sunshine; clean, fresh air; pure water; appropriate physical, mental and emotional activities; and a productive lifestyle) while simultaneously eliminating all harmful factors and influences, the self-constructing, self-regulating, self-repairing qualities of the body are given full rein.

"Whatever Is Natural Is Right"

According to *Health Science*, Sylvester Graham (1794–1851) founded the Hygienic movement in the 1830s. Graham, the originator of the graham cracker, began his career as a Presbyterian minister and temperance lecturer. He held that frequent involuntary discharges of semen presage debility, that the ingestion of "improper" foods or overeating causes seminal discharges, and that

109

masturbation brings on pimples and potentially fatal sores. Graham advocated a vegetarian diet centered on whole grains. In his view, digestion entailed an expenditure of "vital force," diet was a means of economizing this force, and a diet was healthful if it narrowly prompted the digestive organs to function normally.

In *Crusaders for Fitness: The History of American Health Reformers* (1982), James C. Whorton, Ph.D., wrote:

The presupposition that physiology—that is, nature—must be Christian forced Graham and fellow health reformers to perform some tricky mental acrobatics. For in recoiling from the spontaneous expression of appetites and passions, they seemed to be showing distrust of the very nature they professed to worship. The only way out they could find was to deny the naturalness of appetites in the present age by arguing that the pure instincts of original man had been defiled by wrong use of free will and reason. In other paragraphs, however, they make it clear that vitiated appetites could not be subdued except by the exertion of that same slippery will; and natural physiology could be rediscovered only by the exercise of that same unreliable reason.

The Hygienic movement enjoyed considerable popularity, declined, and was revived by Herbert M. Shelton (1895–1985), who cofounded the American Natural Hygiene Society in 1948. "Today," Shelton said in a 1978 *Health Science* interview, "thanks to my untiring effort and the efforts of those who joined me in the work, men that were dead live again, principles that were forgotten have been refurbished, and a whole literature has been salvaged." In a 1982 interview, he claimed he had "brought order out of chaos."

To what principles and to whose order did Shelton allude? In the 1963 edition of *An Introduction to Natural Hygiene*, he stated that a loss of "nerve force" attends sexual orgasm, causing weakness; that people should not indulge in sexual intercourse for pleasure or relief, but only for procreation; that nature or God intended humans to go nude; that "whatever is natural is right"; and that our "natural (unperverted) instincts" can lead us correctly.

Shelton described his educational background in the 1978 interview. At the age of sixteen, having undergone "the usual brainwashing process of the public school system in Greenville, Texas," he "revolted against the whole political, religious, medical, and social system." After serving in the Army during World War I, he obtained his first degree, that of "Doctor of Physiological Therapeutics," from the Macfadden College of Physcultopathy (see previous chapter).

Next, Shelton took a postgraduate course at the Lindlahr College of

Natural Therapeutics in Chicago. The school's founder was Henry Lindlahr, M.D., N.D., an iridology proponent whose medical degree had come from a low-grade medical college. The son of a naturopath, Lindlahr professed that "all disease is caused by something that interferes with, diminishes or disturbs the normal inflow and distribution of vital energy throughout the system."

In *Fads and Quackery in Healing* (1932), Morris Fishbein, M.D., an eminent adversary of quackery, described the *best* of the naturopathy schools then operating between the World Wars:

> Candidates . . . may not be able even to read or write, because preliminary requirements in such schools are given little if any consideration. Although a high-school education may be mentioned as a necessity, its equivalent may be substituted. . . . The professors themselves are without baccalaureate degrees or, in most instances, any other degree of importance.

From Chicago, Shelton went to New York, where, "after nine months of brainwashing," he received doctoral degrees from schools founded by Benedict Lust, one in naturopathy and another in chiropractic. Then he returned to Chicago to do postgraduate work at another chiropractic college, which, Sheldon said, was "accompanied and succeeded by thirty-one months of apprenticeship in four different institutions, where the most valuable thing I learned was what not to do."

The first of Shelton's approximately forty books, *Fundamentals of Nature Cure*, was published in 1920. In 1928, he opened Dr. Shelton's Health School in San Antonio, Texas, which operated at seven different locations until 1981. From 1934 through 1941, Shelton produced a seven-volume series called *The Hygienic System*. In 1949, he launched *Dr. Shelton's Hygienic Review*, a monthly magazine that was published for about forty years.

In 1982, a federal court jury awarded $873,000 to the survivors of William Carlton, a forty-nine-year-old man who had died after undergoing a distilled-water fast for thirty days at Shelton's Health School. An article in the *Los Angeles Daily Journal* stated that Carlton had died of bronchial pneumonia resulting from a weakened condition in which he lost fifty pounds during the last month of his life. The article also noted that he was the sixth person in five years who had died while undergoing "treatment" at the school. Shelton and his associate, chiropractor Vivian V. Vetrano, claimed in their appeal that Carlton had persisted in fasting after Vetrano had advised him to stop. However, the Fifth Circuit Court of Appeals upheld the verdict, and the U.S. Supreme Court declined further review.

Fasting and Food Combining

The American Natural Hygiene Society (ANHS) in Tampa, Florida, is the fountainhead of today's Natural Hygiene activity. Regular ANHS membership costs $25 per year and includes a subscription to *Health Science,* a thirty-two-page bimonthly magazine. A recent mailing stated that ANHS has over eight thousand members. The group has actively promoted certification of "organic" foods and vigorously opposed compulsory immunization and food irradiation.

Each issue of *Health Science* includes a professional referral list. The November/December 1993 issue lists thirty-three people; most are chiropractors, but a few hold a medical, osteopathic, or naturopathic degree. The list includes thirteen "certified" and eight "associate" professional Hygienists in the United States, and others in Australia, Canada, England, Greece, Israel, Japan, and Poland. Certified members include ANHS founders and "subsequent members who have successfully completed an internship (or its equivalent) in Natural Hygiene care with an emphasis on Fasting Supervision."

According to an ANHS brochure:

A thoroughgoing rest, which includes fasting, is the most favorable condition under which an ailing body can purify and repair itself. Fasting is the total abstinence from all liquid and solid foods except distilled water. During a fast the body's recuperative forces are marshaled and all of its energies are directed toward the recharging of the nervous system, the elimination of toxic accumulations, and the repair and rejuvenation of tissue. Stored within each organism's tissues are nutrient reserves which it will use to carry on metabolism and repair work. Until these reserves are depleted, no destruction of healthy tissue or "starvation" can occur.

ANHS publications promote fasting for children as well as for adults. The brochure also states:

Natural Hygiene rejects the use of medications, blood transfusions, radiation, dietary supplements, and any other means employed to treat or "cure" various ailments. These therapies interfere with or destroy vital processes and tissue. Recovery from disease takes place in spite of, and not because of, the drugging and "curing" practices.

Another conspicuous component of Natural Hygiene is food combining. In *Food Combining Made Easy* (a "nutrition classic," according to its cover), Shelton wrote:

To a single article of food that is a starch-protein combination, the body can easily adjust its juices . . . to the digestive requirements of the food.

But when two foods are eaten with different . . . digestive needs, this precise adjustment of juices to requirements becomes impossible.

A Natural Hygienist might claim, for example, that consuming a high-protein food and a high-carbohydrate food at the same meal, at the very least, taxes the body's enzymatic capacity. Researchers revealed the falsity of such ideas more than fifty years ago, but the Hygienic faithful still hold them dear.

In *Food Combining*, Shelton grouped foods "according to their composition and sources of origin": (1) "proteins," including nuts, peanuts, and avocados; (2) "starches" and sweet fruits, including peanuts (again), chestnuts, pumpkin, bananas, and mangoes; (3) "fats," including most nuts (again) and avocados (again); (4) "acid fruits," including citrus fruit and tomatoes; (5) "sub-acid" fruits, including pears and apricots; (6) non-starchy and green vegetables, including lettuce, broccoli, and watercress; and (7) melons, including watermelon, honeydew, and cantaloupe.

Food combining may be on the wane, at least in the Hygienic upper echelon. In the July/August 1993 issue of *Health Science*, professional Hygienist Joel Fuhrman, M.D., states:

> The majority of present-day hygienic physicians do not emphasize food combining as an important component of Natural Hygiene. . . . It is not how you combine your foods that determines your health, rather your overall food choices. . . . Food combining can be made excessively restrictive and, in some cases, may retard growth in infants and children. . . . The majority of people need not be concerned with it if they are generally eating a low protein, low fat, high fiber diet.

Natural Hygiene discourages consumption of meat, poultry, fish, eggs, dairy products, garlic, mustard, radishes, rhubarb, cranberries, maple syrup, honey, salt, pepper, vinegar, margarine, and oils.

Two bestsellers by Harvey and Marilyn Diamond—*Fit for Life* (1985) and *Living Health* (1987)—sparked a renaissance for Natural Hygiene. Harvey Diamond received his "Ph.D. in nutritional science" from the American College of Health Science, a correspondence school in Texas that has offered—under a half-dozen names—courses detailing the views of its administrator, T.C. Fry. Marilyn Diamond holds a "master's degree" from the school, which is now called Health Excellence Systems. However, it has never been accredited or legally authorized to grant degrees. In 1986, Mr. Fry agreed to a permanent injunction barring him from representing his enterprise as a college or granting any more "degrees" or "academic credits" without authorization from the Texas Department of Higher Education. According to his paperback *Laugh Your Way to Health* (1991), Fry did not complete high school, but attended college for three months—then dropped out "because they had nothing of significance to teach." The Diamonds quote him in *Living Health*: "On the day of reckoning, I doubt we will be judged by what certificates we have on the wall, but rather by the scars incurred in the battle for humanity."

AHNS basks in the *Fit for Life* furor to this day. In the November/ December 1993 issue of *Health Science*, the society's executive director, James Michael Lennon, states:

> A new day has dawned for Natural Hygiene and the American Natural Hygiene Society. It is a bright, shining day.
>
> After 150 years of relative obscurity, Natural Hygiene is now recognized as a major force for change in health care. . . .
>
> What is creating this new interest and recognition? . . . First and foremost is the extraordinary attention that was focused on Natural Hygiene when Harvey and Marilyn Diamond's *Fit for Life* books appeared. These books reached over 11 million readers initially and are still reaching people around the world with translations into many languages.
>
> Another important factor is the growth of the American Natural Hygiene Society, which has tripled in size in the last ten years. . . .
>
> While the teachings of Natural Hygiene have changed very little in recent years, the way they are presented has changed dramatically. There has also been a change of emphasis.
>
> *Fit for Life* was the first book to present Natural Hygiene as a happy, enjoyable, health-building tool, available for use by intelligent people who want the best for themselves and their families. In addition to the upbeat mood, this book was a "starter book," designed to help as wide an audience as possible. It did not try to present Natural Hygiene in its purest theoretical form all at once. It set the stage for additional books to be written.

The Bottom Line

The mainstays of "natural healing" are wishful thinking, superstition, empiricism, guesswork, and enmity toward scientific healthcare. Rituals and proselytism communicate its "spiritual" basis. Although fresh air, exercise, and consumption of fresh fruits and vegetables are important components of healthy living, the Hygienists' overall dietary regimen and their avoidance of medical care are foolish and potentially harmful.

Part IV

Physical Cultism

10

"Hands-On Healing"

In "alternative" healthcare, "bodywork" is an umbrella term for many treatments that involve touching, manipulation, and/or exercise of the body and, in most cases, supposed alignment of the body's "energy field" or removal of blockages to the flow of "energy." Bodywork encompasses massage therapy, body-centered psychotherapy, and touch therapy. "Touch therapy" and "touch healing" are generic terms for the laying on of hands and its variants, including OMEGA, reiki, and therapeutic touch.

Unlike scientific physical therapists, proponents recommend bodywork for many health problems beyond pain, physical dysfunction, and physical injury. Not all forms of bodywork are supernaturalistic, but most are unscientific. Supernaturalistic forms include actualism bodywork, acupuncture, acu-yoga, amma therapy, aromatherapy, *Bindegewebsmassage*, biodynamic massage, bioenergetics, body harmony, bodywork tantra, *chi nei tsang*, fundamentalist chiropractic, core energetics, craniosacral therapy, *do-in*, Esalen massage, the hakomi method, hatha yoga, Hawaiian temple bodywork, healing light kung fu, holotropic therapy, *jin shin do*, *jin shin jyutsu*, josephing, *kum nye*, life impressions bodywork, lomi-lomi, manual organ stimulation therapy (MOST), marma therapy, the metamorphic technique, moxibustion, Ohashiatsu, ortho-bionomy, phoenix rising yoga therapy, polarity balancing, the radiance technique, radix, rebirthing, reflexology, Reichian massage, reiki, rolfing, the Rubenfeld synergy method, shiatsu, sotai, Tibetan pulsing, Touch for Health, Trager, and Chinese Qigong massage (including amma, *tui na*, and *dian xue*).

In *World Medicine: The East West Guide to Healing Your Body*

117

(1993), Tom Monte and associates state: "Since the 1960s, healing touch emerged as if from below ground in the form of a variety of bodywork therapies. . . . While the techniques differ somewhat, the basic principles are essentially the same: the body, mind, and spirit are a unified entity, and by healing the body, one frees the mind and spirit of conflicts, distress, and illness."

This chapter describes my experiences with eight types of bodywork. In each case, I informed the practitioner that I was investigating different methods for the purpose of writing a book.

Rolfing

Rolfing is a deep-massage technique of "muscular realignment" promoted mainly for back and neck problems. However, proponents also claim it facilitates weight loss, relieves anxiety, and increases stamina and self-esteem. Ida P. Rolf, Ph.D. (1896–1979), an organic chemist who had studied yoga and chiropractic, developed the method in New York in the 1930s. Rolf compared her technique to "rebuilding a sagging or bulging brick wall, rather than trying to prop it up by artificial means." The Rolf Institute in Boulder, Colorado, founded in 1971, quotes her in a pamphlet: "Rolfers make a life study of relating bodies and their fields to the earth and its gravity field, and we so organize the body that the gravity field can reinforce the body's energy field." Rolfers adjust the massage when they supposedly detect areas of "energy imbalance" within the body.

The standard rolfing series consists of ten sessions, each lasting from sixty to ninety minutes and costing between $60 and $100. Practitioners focus each session on a different body part. According to rolfing theory, the body may become rigid because of emotional trauma. Proponents claim that one's posture reveals past traumatic experiences, that rolfing effects emotional and "energetic" release, and that this alleged release restores the flow of "vital energy" and integrates mind and body.

In the March/April 1993 issue of *Natural Health*, Mirka Knaster describes a rolfer's client: "Rolfing is helping her lift up and out of her collapsed body structure." But during one session, writes Knaster, this client began to "shiver uncontrollably." Her trembling increased, her jaw quivered, and she whimpered like a child. Knaster ascribes the client's behavior to the "sudden evocation" of a "body memory." This concept is based on a theory formulated by psychoanalyst Wilhelm Reich (see Chapter 3). The theory holds that muscles and connective tissue store memories as "undischarged energy" (orgone) and that therapists can access this "energy" by massaging the patient.

Before being rolfed at Newlife Expo '93 in New York City, I had never undergone a professional massage or any other kind of bodywork. The cost of the session was a dollar a minute, with a fifteen-minute minimum. Before he began, Chuck Carpenter, the "certified advanced rolfer," inquired if anything was wrong with my body. I replied that I was not aware of any physical problem at the moment, but that I sometimes had mild pain in the lower part of my back, probably due to sporadic weightlifting. He asked me to remove my shirt and observed me standing. Then I lay on the table and he asked me to turn my head far to each side. He noted that it was more difficult for me to turn my head to the left than to the right. Mr. Carpenter confined his manipulation to my upper back, upper arms, and neck, even though I had no neck problem and had not reported one. He said that the goal of future treatment would be to align my collarbones. Overall, the experience was pleasant. The treatment felt like a slow process of molding. But, while pressure was the principal sensation, I also felt dull pain and prickling. Mr. Carpenter said that rolfing is painful to some clients. In any case, the sensations I experienced were ephemeral and unremarkable, and there were no aftereffects—or, at least, no pleasant ones. Although I had not lifted weights in more than forty-eight hours, a little later that day my lower back began to hurt.

I informed Mr. Carpenter that I was a skeptic engaged in an investigation of vitalistic "healing" methods. He affirmed that "energy flows through the body" but added that this was not a premise of rolfing. He said that the association of rolfing with vitalistic concepts may have resulted from its early affiliation with humanistic psychology. Nevertheless, he conferred plausibility to the notion that "energy pathways" run through connective tissue, and stated that sometimes clients "release" painful memories during a session, such as of being abused in childhood. When I expressed disbelief in "energy pathways," Mr. Carpenter cited the Chinese medicine episode of "Healing and the Mind with Bill Moyers" (see Chapter 4).

It seems that whether rolfing is discomforting or dangerous depends mainly on the personal technique and zealousness of the practitioner. *The Encyclopedia of Alternative Health Care* (1989) describes an incomplete session so painful that the client had to resign his job.

Polarity Therapy

In May and June 1993, I experienced six other forms of bodywork—polarity therapy, *jin shin do*, shiatsu, foot reflexology, Swedish massage, and craniosacral balancing—at the New York Open Center, Inc., in Manhattan's Soho district. The Open Center, founded in 1984, describes itself as "a non-profit educational and multi-cultural center offering programs designed to heal the body, nourish the soul and awaken the spirit." It offers more than nine hundred seminars annually in such subjects as acupressure, anthroposophy, *A Course in Miracles*, "holistic" aromatherapy, BRETH, craniosacral therapy, *ki* breathing, foot reflexology, herbalism, holotropic breathwork, homeopathy, *I Ching*, "imaginal medicine," "kundalini awakening," marma therapy, meditation, past-life therapy, psychic self-defense, Qigong therapy, Rubenfeld synergy, sacred dance, shamanism, shiatsu, synchronicity, the tarot, therapeutic touch, Touch for Health, and yoga. Its Summer 1993 catalog cited Eisenberg's "unconventional medicine" survey (see Chapter 4) and the PBS series "Healing and the Mind with Bill Moyers." As a package, the six one-hour sessions cost $275. The fee for individual sessions would have been $55 per hour. All of them took place in a comfortably large room.

Polarity therapy encompasses counseling, craniosacral balancing (see below), "energetic nutrition," guided imagery, polarity yoga (polarity exercise), and reflexology (see below). Its originator, Austrian-born Randolph Stone (1890–1982), was a naturopath, chiropractor, and osteopath who retired to live in India in 1973. In *Your Healing Hands: The Polarity Experience* (1984), Richard Gordon states:

> Life-force flows through the body as if it were following an invisible circulatory system, charging every cell in its path. This current of energy can become weakened and partially blocked due to stress. . . . In polarity energy balancing, physical and nonphysical touch techniques are used to send energy through the entire system to open up the blocked points. This reestablishes the proper flow and alignment of life-force throughout the body.

Polarity theory holds that the top and right side of the body have a positive charge, and that the feet and the left side of the body have a negative charge. Thus, practitioners place their right hand (+) on "negatively charged" parts of the client's body, and their left hand (-) on "positively charged" parts.

My polarity session included craniosacral balancing, foot reflexology, and conversation. The practitioner, Ann Seham, said she knew Chuck Carpenter, who had rolfed me at Newlife Expo '93. She described his style as "mild." Fully clothed except for shoes, I lay on my back on a cushioned table. A scented candle was lit. Ms. Seham performed only five notable actions: She began by moving my head gently from the middle of the table toward one side, then the other, and repeated the sequence several times. She lifted one of my arms, told me to relax it, and held it awhile. She placed one of her arms below my sacrum and the other on my waist and gently rocked me. She massaged my feet, and she stroked the underside of my legs with her fingers. For most of the hour, Ms. Seham simply applied finger-pressure to various areas of my body, especially to the skull and the back of my neck.

Jin Shin Do

Jin shin do is a system of acupressure based on the book *Way of the Compassionate Spirit,* acupuncture theory, Taoist philosophy, and Reichian theory (see Glossary and Chapter 3). Iona Marsaa Teeguarden, author of *Acupressure Way of Health* (1978) and *Joy of Feeling: Bodymind Acupressure* (1987), developed *jin shin do* in the 1970s. Practitioners determine which parts of the body are "tense." According to *jin shin do* theory, stressful experiences cause the building of tension at certain "acupoints." To "balance" the "energy" of the body, practitioners hold the "tense" part with one hand and supposedly stimulate a series of acupoints with the other. Proponents recommend *jin shin do* for allergies, bedwetting, constipation, nocturnal coughing, ear infections, lung congestion, nosebleeds, hyperkinesis in children, and other conditions.

My *jin shin do* session, which took place in the same room at the Open Center, was more stimulating than my polarity experience. As I again lay on my back fully clothed except for shoes, the practitioner, Elana Sheridan, applied finger-pressure to my back, chest, face, and pelvis. Toward the end of the session, she repeatedly slapped the top and sole of each foot. However, for much of the hour, she simply held either foot with one hand and, with the other, applied pressure to areas on the upper part of my body. She suggested that the heart is the seat of the emotions. Ms. Sheridan finished with ceremonial movements of her arms and hands. She explained that although both *jin shin do* and shiatsu are variants of acupressure, the former is based on Taoism—yin and yang, the dark and the light.

Shiatsu

Shiatsu is a Japanese form of "therapeutic" massage in which practitioners apply pressure with the palms and four fingers of each hand to those areas of the body used in acupuncture. The goal of shiatsu is to promote health by increasing the flow of *ki* in the body. It is based on both acupuncture theory and amma, an early form of oriental "therapeutic" massage. There are three major types of shiatsu: shiatsu massage, which is based largely on amma; acupressure, a strictly manual variant of acupuncture; and Zen shiatsu. The late Shizuto

Masunaga developed Zen shiatsu. Unlike the other types, it incorporates *kyo-jitsu*—the localizing of "imbalances" of *ki* by palpation (touch). In Zen shiatsu, practitioners apply less pressure than in shiatsu massage or acupressure.

Simpson Wong was my shiatsu practitioner at the Open Center. He stated that he was a Malaysian, had graduated from a shiatsu school in his native country, and had lived in the United States for several years since entering on a tourist visa. He described shiatsu as a "spiritual" method and said that one of its goals is to promote self-healing. Mr. Wong asked me to remove only my shoes and belt and to lie on a futon in the middle of the floor. He asked whether I had any physical or emotional problems. I replied that I had thinning hair and gum disease. He suggested that I apply aloe vera to my scalp to increase hair growth. Mr. Wong rarely spoke during the session; generally, he did so only in response to questions. Before applying finger-pressure to certain areas, he applied pressure with his palms to "warm" them. He prepared each leg for finger pressure by folding it toward my chest with his shoulder. He also massaged the soles of my feet with his fists and my scalp and face with his fingers.

Reflexology

"Reflexology" is a generic term that refers to the stimulation of specific areas ("reflex points") under the skin. William H. Fitzgerald, M.D., a specialist in diseases of the ear, nose, and throat, introduced reflexology in the United States in 1913 as zone therapy. Fitzgerald divided the human body into ten zones and taught that "bioelectrical" energy flowed through these zones to "reflex points" in the hands and feet. His method, which was also called zonotherapy, involved the fastening of wire springs around toes. Eunice D. Ingham, an American, further developed reflexology in the 1930s and 1940s, concentrating on the feet. It is purportedly useful in assessing and improving the function of specific body parts. Proponents hold that all bodily organs have corresponding external "reflex points" (particularly on the feet) and that manipulation of these can enhance the flow of "energy." They localize "reflex points" not only on the feet, but on the scalp, ears, face, nose, tongue, neck, back, arms, wrists, hands, abdomen, and legs.

Reflexology tools include clothespins, combs, rubber balls, rubber bands, tongue depressors, wire brushes, and special devices, including: the "reflex foot massager," the "reflex roller massager," the "reflex hand probe," and "reflex clamps." Proponents recommend reflexology for acne, alcoholism, asthma, bedwetting, constipation, diabetes, fatigue, hypertension, kidney stones, migraines, multiple sclerosis, pyorrhea (gum inflammation), shingles, sinus congestion, whiplash, and diseases of the liver and pancreas.

Body Reflexology: Healing at Your Fingertips (1983) includes a chapter titled "Diet, Vitamins, and Reflexology." In it, Mildred Carter, a former student of William Fitzgerald, recommended brewer's yeast, blackstrap molasses, lecithin, and yogurt as "wonder foods." She stated: "Any cooked food is dead food. . . . Live food has a vibratory rate that generates life! . . . It takes a living thing to keep another living thing alive." A 1993 mailing from the book's publisher, Parker Publishing Company of West Nyack, New York, contained more than twenty testimonials and stated:

> Not only does new Body Reflexology let you cure the worst illnesses safely and permanently, *it can even work to reverse the aging process,* Carter says. Say goodbye to age lines, dry skin, brown spots, blemishes—with Body Reflexology you can actually give yourself an *at-home facelift* with *no* discomfort or disfiguring surgery.

Cathy Allen, my reflexologist at the Open Center, said she taught reflexology out of the Swedish Institute (see below) as a partner in Laura Norman and Associates. This firm's advertisement in the April/May 1993 issue of *Free Spirit* claimed that foot reflexology can "cleanse the body of toxins," "revitalize energies," "balance the system," strengthen the immune system, facilitate weight loss, and enhance creativity and productivity.

On a table in the same room with the candle lit, I lay barefoot on my back, listening to an audiotape that included much chanting. Ms. Allen performed foot reflexology. She applied lotion to my feet before massaging them. Although she emphasized that she routinely "backed away" from voicing a diagnosis, she did say that I had "some tightness" in my intestines. She also remarked that many reflexologists have no compunctions about rendering diagnoses.

Swedish Massage

Swedish massage is the most commonly practiced form of bodywork in Western countries. Proponents ascribe the development of the basis for the modern system to Peter Hendrik (Per Henrick) Ling (1776–1839) of Sweden. Ling was a fencing master, physiologist, and poet. His method was called the "Ling system" or the "Swedish movement treatment." Dr. S.W. Mitchell introduced it in the United States. Swedish massage is based on scientific anatomy, focused on soft tissue, and often vigorous. Its goal is to improve the circulation of the blood and lymph. Proponents recommend Swedish massage for AIDS, arthritis, back pain, bronchial asthma, constipation, emphysema, neck pain, pneumonia, headaches, heart disease, hypertension, indigestion, multiple sclerosis, quitting smoking, sprains, and insomnia. Although Swedish massage is not inherently supernaturalistic, the claims made for it are sometimes overblown and it is apparently an important seedbed for supernaturalistic forms of bodywork. For example, the Swedish Institute, Inc., in New York City's borough of Manhattan, offers training not only in Swedish massage but in Qigong, rebirthing, reiki, rolfing, shiatsu, *tui na*, Chinese herbalism, color healing, and a variant of bioenergetics. The institute, founded in 1916, has been accredited since 1981 by the Career College Association, which is not a regional accrediting agency.

Swedish massage consists of five basic movements: rhythmic stroking, kneading, friction, percussion, and vibration ("shaking"). Practitioners treat the back, arms, hands, abdomen, feet, legs, head, and face.

Barbara Rice, my masseuse, was a graduate of the Swedish Institute. When she began, I lay on my stomach wearing only briefs, with my face in a "face cradle" attached to the end of the table. She applied canola oil to my back and used both her hands and forearms. Later, I lay on my back. I was often somewhat uncomfortable during the massage, and my trapezius muscles (which span the areas between the back of the neck and each shoulder) became sore.

Craniosacral Balancing

Craniosacral balancing allegedly involves manually aligning skull bones—which, in fact, are fused and not "adjustable." The purported goal of such "manipulation" is to remove impediments to the patient's "energy." The therapist holds the skull in his hand and supposedly attunes himself to the patient's "rhythm." Proponents claim that about 95 percent of people suffer from misalignment of cranial bones, which, they say, causes toothaches, migraines, and neurological disturbances. Dr. William Garner Sutherland developed cranial osteopathy over a thirty-year period in the early 1900s. Sutherland was a student of Dr. Andrew Taylor Still (1828–1917), the founder of osteopathy. Still asserted that God had revealed osteopathy to him. He taught that removal of structural defects enabled the body's "life force" to create health.

According to cranial osteopathy, movements of the skull bones cause movements of the sacrum and vice versa. In *Osteopathy: The Illustrated Guide*

(1989), Stephen Sandler, D.O., explains: "Osteopaths who have studied and specialized in this system maintain that palpation on the skull and sacrum can pick up a rhythmic pulsation distinct from the respiratory rhythm or heartbeat and pulse of the blood. This pulsation is the reverberation of the cerebrospinal fluid, which bathes both the brain and the spinal cord." Derivatives of Sutherland's approach are utilized by chiropractors, dentists, and other practitioners, who may refer to their work as cranial osteopathy, cranial therapy, and/or craniosacral therapy. The New York Wellness Bodywork Center™ describes craniosacral theory in a flyer:

> At the core of all the body's rhythms is a subtle wave-like pulse which moves through the fluid surrounding the brain and spinal cord. Constrictions in the membranes that surround this fluid can affect the transmission of this pulse throughout our body's energy fields and structures. Gentle touch and manipulations are synchronized with the cranial rhythms to allow the release of these constrictions.

Ruth Kaciak, my "craniosacral balancer," asked if I had any problem she should concentrate on. I replied that I had gum disease. Ms. Kaciak said she usually blends craniosacral balancing with other forms of bodywork, but she agreed to perform "straight" craniosacral work during the session. As I lay on my back on the table, she passed her hands over me without touching. She said that advanced craniosacral balancers need not touch the body. "Everything can be done in the aura," she explained. Some practitioners, she added, use craniosacral balancing only as a diagnostic method. (In the world of the occult, the aura is an envelope or "spiritual skin" of "subtle energy" that surrounds magnets, crystals, and all living bodies. Supposedly, human auras are visible to clairvoyants and reveal the passions and vices of the soul.)

Ms. Kaciak professed to work "on the emotional plane." She noted a "vibration" in the middle of my chest and said it related to the "heart chakra." She also claimed to detect "emotional stuff" in my right hip. However, she decided that there was a "real smoothness" to my "energy" and pronounced me emotionally balanced.

She said that craniosacral balancing is a way of releasing "blocked emotional energy" and that its goal is "to free the craniosacral system." She further stated:

> I don't think it's a matter of modality. It's a matter of the relationship between the client and the practitioner. . . . I think that whatever is needed usually appears. . . . I work intuitively. . . . Your intention is everything in healing. . . . [Bodywork is] an art form. It's who the person is, rather than the technique that they're using. . . . A lot of craniosacral stuff goes back to birth trauma.

Ms. Kaciak asserted that bodywork basically involves finding a "blockage" or "deficiency" of energy and correcting it. However, she opined that "the altered state" is "the other major component of the bodywork experience." "I go into an altered state, too," she said. (During the second half of the session, she appeared to be in somewhat of a trance.) Ms. Kaciak said that craniosacral balancers do not necessarily seek to relieve the problems their clients report. She explained: "It may be good that they're dying. . . . Maybe they need that knee problem for some other reason." According to Ms. Kaciak, a need for self-development may be the inconspicuous "reason" for—or "message" of— an illness.

Ms. Kaciak applied pressure with her fingers to points on the right side of my body from my hip upward. Then she lifted my head slightly and turned it slowly several times right and left. She asserted that cranial bones can become "jammed" or "pulled out of alignment." She also lightly moved her fingertips on my forehead and other parts of my face and placed her hands below my waist. The session reminded me of my *jin shin do* experience.

The Alexander Technique

The Alexander technique is a murky "body/mind" method focused on posture improvement. Proponents claim that maintaining alignment of the head, neck, and back leads to optimum overall physical functioning. They further claim that it is useful in the treatment of a variety of diseases, including asthma, hypertension, peptic ulcer disease, and ulcerative colitis. Frederick Matthias Alexander (1869–1955), an Australian Shakespearean actor, developed the method at the turn of the century. Although his original purpose was to assist voice projection, Alexander concluded that faulty posture was responsible for diverse symptoms. He postulated that habitual unbalanced movement affects the functioning of the entire body— implying that postures entail behavior patterns and that bad postural habits can distort one's personality. Alexander further postulated that there was one basic movement—the maximum lengthening of the spine—from which all proper bodily movements flowed. This he termed the "primary control."

According to *Body Awareness in Action: A Study of the Alexander Technique* (1979), Alexander held that heredity was a negligible determinant of behavior, that it could be "practically eradicated" in the "vast majority of cases," and that the "capacity for good and evil is very great" within hereditary limits. In one of his four books, Alexander stated that, in a sense, his method embraced all religions. He described the "Great Origin of the Universe" as an "all-wise and invisible Authority"—a "high power within the soul of man" that enables behavior subordinate to itself.

Teachers of the technique convey it by manually applying gentle pressure to various parts of the student's body and simultaneously repeating key phrases. The student usually is seated or lies on a table. Sessions—which proponents call lessons—typically last from thirty minutes to an hour and cost between $20 and $75 each. One teacher has distributed a flyer titled "Bone Meditation," which states: "By separating the bones from one another, you can feel energy flow through and out the finger tips." The technique is popular with performing artists.

In May 1993, I experienced the method at the Manhattan Center for the Alexander Technique in New York City. Lessons are between forty-five minutes and an hour long and cost $35. Lawrence Smith, my teacher, was a former dancer. His posture was impeccable. He described himself as a "hardcore atheist" and said he didn't believe in the existence of the soul. He also stated that the Alexander technique tended to become "diluted" with spiritualistic theories and methods. However, he said he believed in the existence of *chi* and cited Master Shir's "demonstrations" of external Qigong on "Healing and the Mind with Bill Moyers" (see Chapter 4).

Smith likened F.M. Alexander's basic "discovery"—the "primary control"—to a "master reflex." He stated that it was unwise to interfere with it and that one could minimize interference by learning to inhibit one's immediate response to stress. Inefficient movement of the neck supposedly manifests interference with the so-called primary control. Smith explained that, generally, to "short-circuit" this unconscious habit, one must ascertain what stimulus had originally provoked the allegedly unhealthy neck movement.

My lesson took place in a large room filled with daylight. The room contained a table; two firm, comfortable armless chairs; and several firm, round stools. At Smith's request, I sat on a stool. He noted that if my manner of sitting was habitual, I was probably interfering with the "primary control." I rose and sat down again. Smith asked me why I contracted my neck in the process of sitting down. I responded that perhaps the contraction was due to uncertainty regarding the location of the seat. "I think you hit on something," he conceded. After evaluating my sitting style, Smith gave me simultaneous manual and verbal directions on how to sit down and rise properly. His hands were around my neck as I repeatedly rose and sat down. When he told me not to respond with my neck muscles to his manipulation, I countered that the reaction may be one of self-preservation. He stated that the "antigravity response" is one of "extension" rather than "hardening." "My job," he explained, "is to point things out to you and to try to guide you out of contraction." He said that the Alexander technique typically causes considerable discomfort in persons with "strong habitual patterns." During the latter part of the lesson, I lay on the table with my head upon two paperbacks. Meanwhile, Smith repeatedly pulled my neck and limbs, purportedly to lengthen my body.

A Mixed Bag

Bodywork is a mixed bag. Its many forms range from the secular (e.g., rolfing, Swedish massage, and the Alexander technique) to the spiritual (e.g., polarity therapy and *jin shin do*). Some practitioners render vague or weird "diagnoses," while other practitioners appear to recognize their limitations. Massage of specific parts of the body may relieve symptoms in the area massaged, but the idea that applying pressure to one area of the body can remedy a problem in a distant area is unfounded. The Alexander technique may, with perseverance, improve posture, but craniosacral balancing, which is anatomically impossible, is futile.

The next chapter focuses on a quasireligious form of bodywork. Chapter 12 covers distinctly psychological forms, and Chapter 13 deals with chiropractic supernaturalism.

11

Reiki

Reiki, a variant of the laying on of hands, is not only a type of bodywork but a form of energy field work. Energy field work overlaps with bodywork and encompasses all methods involving aura analysis and aura balancing, with or without touch. One practitioner I contacted, whose fee was $90 per two-hour session, described reiki as "a modality based more on energy than on pressure." A flyer from the Loving Touch Center of New York describes it as a 2,500-year-old "natural Tibetan healing art" that is "not a religion" and "does not require a belief system to work." Proponents recommend reiki as a complement to acupressure, acupuncture, the Alexander technique, chiropractic, homeopathy, polarity balancing, rolfing, therapeutic touch, and yoga.

Keepers of the "Sacred System"

In the United States, the three dominant reiki organizations are the American Reiki Master Association (ARMA) in Lake City, Florida; the Radiance Technique Association International, Inc., in St. Petersburg, Florida; and the Reiki Alliance, which has offices in Cataldo, Idaho, and Amsterdam, the Netherlands. The Reiki Alliance's March 1993 membership list included 515 people in twenty-five states and twenty-eight other countries. In August 1993, ARMA had thirty-one "master teachers" in the United States, Canada, Mexico, Central America, and Switzerland. The *Journal of the American Reiki Master Association* promotes nutritional supplementation, aromatherapy, astrology, aura balancing, chakra balancing, crystal therapy, guided visualization, the

129

kofutu system, mahikari, numerology, "psychic prayer," radionics, reflexology, shiatsu, tarot training, and urine therapy. Rev. Arthur L. Robertson, Ph.D., founded ARMA in 1988. His business card designates him a "sacred scientist." In response to my telephone request for information, Robertson mailed me a stapled handbook that included the notice:

> THIS MANUAL CONTAINS THE SACRED AND HIDDEN SECRETS OF REIKI. DO NOT LEAVE YOUR MANUAL LAYING AROUND WHERE OTHERS CAN FIND IT AND READ IT. THIS IS A 'SACRED SYSTEM,' AND SHOULD BE GUARDED AND PROTECTED AS SUCH.

ARMA is an "outreach" of a church called the Omega Dawn Sanctuary of Healing Arts, which shares ARMA's address. Through this church, Robertson markets the "Antahkarana Master Frequency Unit," a "perpetual self-empowered broadcaster." He claims that the joint use of three of these units effects remission from AIDS in about an hour and a half. The device allegedly relieves other illnesses—such as Alzheimer's disease, cancer, and multiple sclerosis—"virtually instantaneously." The large model costs $375 and the small one $150. Other "powerful healing devices" range in price from $49 to $375.

Reiki's Legendary Origin

Mikao Usui (1802–1883), the head of a Christian seminary for boys and later a Zen Buddhist monk, founded reiki as a religious movement in Japan in the late nineteenth century. Usui held a doctorate in theology from the University of Chicago. "Reiki" combines two Japanese words: *rei* and *ki*. Interpretations of the word *rei* include "cosmic, universal energy," "ghost," "soul," "spirit," "spiritual body," and "free passage." The word *ki* signifies both breath and attention ("mental force"). *Ki* is an alleged original, fundamental, supernatural, governable, creative "energy of being" concentrated in the abdomen. "Reiki" refers both to "spirit energy" and to a method that is largely a variant of aura balancing and the laying on of hands.

The highlight of Usui's legendary discovery—or rediscovery—of reiki was a paranormal experience. Usui fasted and meditated for twenty days on a "holy mountain" near Kyoto. Before sunrise on the twenty-first day, he saw a "light" speeding toward him. The light struck him in the middle of his forehead, opening his "third eye"—the *ajna* chakra, supposedly the human body's highest source of power. In *Reiki Plus Natural Healing* (1991), reiki master Reverend David G. Jarrell writes:

> He thought he had died and had ascended into heaven. He had never

before been in such a euphoric state. His entire field of vision was a rainbow of color. Out of the rainbow came bubbles of gold, white, blue, and violet. Each of the different bubbles contained symbolic messages. A voice said, "These are the keys to healing; learn them, do not forget them; and, do not allow them to be lost."

Golden Sanskrit letters in the light—the "keys to healing" to which Jarrell refers—supposedly constitute the basis of reiki.

"Attunements"

In *The Reiki Touch: A Reiki Handbook* (1990), reiki master Judy-Carol Stewart describes the "energy" of reiki as "pure God-force" that "flows from the universe into the crown chakra, the throat chakra, and the heart chakra, then out the arms and hands." This "love healing force," she continues, "has divine intelligence and will seek its own path in discovering and fulfilling the body's requirement." The method involves touching parts of the body and "brushing" its alleged "aura" with the hands. The apparent aim is to transfer "universal life force energy" and thus effect healing and harmony. Stewart distinguishes between "Reiki I energy" and "Reiki II energy" and states that practitioners can use the latter for absent healing.

The practitioner or "reiki channel" supposedly visualizes Sanskrit symbols. Students undergo one to seven stages—rites wherein they purportedly receive "attunements" from reiki masters. Some "attunements" allegedly link the student to the "universal life-force energy"; others supposedly intensify the "energy." Reiki masters may administer "attunements" by tracing the Sanskrit symbols on the student's head and on areas corresponding to chakras. In the May/June 1992 issue of *Natural Health*, senior editor Bill Thomson reported that rituals at the first three levels cost hundreds of dollars each and that, in 1985, the Radiance Technique Association International (then called the American International Reiki Association) charged $5,000 for fourth-degree "attunements." The Center for Reiki Training, in Southfield, Michigan, offers a two-day Reiki III "intensive" for $600 that covers "how to give yourself attunements" and "how to send attunements to others at a distance."

There are different schools of reiki. On the telephone, one reiki teacher told me that reiki had proliferated so that "now everybody and their dog is a reiki master." She also said that many teachers have adulterated the Usui system by not discriminating between the traditional system and their personal judgments. One prominent school is that of the radiance technique (TRT). TRT's leading promoter is Barbara Weber Ray, Ph.D., author of *The 'Reiki' Factor in the*

Radiance Technique (1992). The book's cover describes Ray as a "professional, licensed astrologer," a "practicing clairvoyant," and an "especially gifted reader of the I Ching." Her doctorate is in humanities. She states that TRT is not a religion, cult, belief system, or form of psychic healing. In the Summer 1987 issue of *The Radiance Technique*® *Journal,* she stated: "The inherent *purpose* of The Radiance Technique is to give direct access to transcendental, universal, Light-energy. This transcendental energy science accesses a total, non-partial, non-fragmented, universal cosmic order of energy which is *not at all* the same as non-universal, partial, lower vibrational energies which are commonly familiar to us." In *The Official Handbook of The Radiance Technique* (1987), she declares:

> In 1980, there began to occur some progressive fragmentation and confusion in thinking and understanding about how this science is actually activated and transmitted. This fragmentation occurred in that moment when a person *without* the real capacity of being an actual Fifth Degree of this system, without the knowledge of the correct Attunement Process which would also have to be properly interconnected with the whole, began randomly "making teachers." Using parts disconnected from the whole system and making up formulas and methods which were never related to the activation of the energy of this system is a process that has no relation whatever to this system rediscovered by Dr. Usui. It was "something" other than this science. And those individuals had none of the ingredients necessary for the orderly process of this science to occur. WHATEVER THAT "SOMETHING" ELSE WAS, THEY CALLED IT "reiki."

Ray's *Official Handbook* includes drawings that clarify positions for "treating" cats, dogs, and plants with reiki.

The Reiki Handbook (1992) by Larry E. Arnold and Sandra K. Nevius features a "Glossary of Ailments." This provides special instructions for treating nearly a hundred health problems, including brain damage, broken bones, cancer, diabetes, epilepsy, gallstones, hemophilia, radiation sickness, sickle cell anemia, and venereal diseases. The *Handbook* also includes "reiki recipes" for cornmeal bread, wheat-germ zucchini bread, "reiki slaw," soymilk, and a "blood replenisher."

ARMA's first-degree reiki manual states:

> When reiki fails, the willingness of the client to be healed is simply an "alibi." Subconsciously the client does not want to be healed or made healthy again. Many people cling to an illness, which they obviously feel is an advantage to them in some way. With many this is a way to get attention and sympathy. . . .

At times the person has not yet had the time to learn the "lesson" taught by the illness, and therefore they have to go on with the illness for a while. This illness may prevent the client from breaking laws of nature and doing harm to themselves in some way. . . .

Other times a client will come in to you in order to prove to themselves, and also to you, that a method such as Reiki has no possible effect upon any condition whatsoever. They will lie upon the treatment table full of tension, fear, doubt, and skepticism, they resist every flow of energy and pleasant sensation. They also are fighting any kind of inner change, and resist any kind of harmony within the body temple.

The "Healing Circle"

On the evening of June 3, 1993, I attended a two-hour "healing circle" meeting at the Loving Touch Center of New York. Loving Touch is an interfaith church whose headquarters is on the second floor of a seven-story building in midtown Manhattan. The center has branches in Long Island and Albany, New York; Ashland, Oregon; Durango, Colorado; and Hollywood, Florida. It offers Reiki I, Reiki II, and "advanced practitioner" seminars, each of which covers two consecutive days, totals sixteen hours, and results in certification. Reiki master Reverend Samuel Strauss, a "holistic practitioner," founded the center and directs it with his wife, Anita, who is also a minister. A flyer states:

> The reason for our becoming a Ministry was to serve humankind and our alumni. As Interfaith Ministers you will be able to gain entrance to hospitals at almost anytime. As a Spiritualist Church we have written into our purpose for being hand-on faith healing. The designation we give our ministers is "Ministers of Spiritual Healing."

On May 31, 1993 (Memorial Day), I called the center to request a referral to a reiki practitioner. Anita Strauss answered the phone and asked me if any particular physical, mental, or spiritual problem had prompted my call. I replied that I was primarily interested in learning about reiki. She later suggested I attend one of the center's free "healing circle" meetings. Addressing my desire to experience a standard form of reiki, Ms. Strauss said that "recipients" usually lie on tables during reiki sessions but sit in chairs at the meetings. After I met her, she told me that the center occasionally offers workshops on methods that reiki practitioners can "add to their bag of tricks." Such offerings have covered aromatherapy, astrology, aura analysis, the cabala, crystal therapy, graphology, "herbology," hypnotherapy, meditation, numerology, nutrition, palmistry, "psychic awareness," reflexology, the tarot, and yoga.

The above-mentioned flyer describes Ms. Strauss:

Having had a serious life threatening illness 10 years ago, Anita has learned to heal her body with nutrition, exercise and positive thinking. Since then, she has studied alternative methods for healing. Today Anita is certified in the ancient healing arts of Aromatherapy, Reflexology and Massage Therapy. As a Reiki Master, she combines all of her modalities using Reiki as the Universal "glue."

Before the meeting began, Strauss related how she had become a reiki practitioner: In the 1980s, while employed as a medical technologist at a Florida hospital, she received inpatient treatment for bleeding ulcers. During her hospital stay, she decided to quit this job to relieve stress. After discharge, however, she not only resumed working full-time but enrolled full-time at a massage school. Six months later she graduated and began working part-time as a massage therapist. Shortly afterward, nagging symptoms prompted her to try reiki. After three sessions, she decided to become a practitioner. She met her husband, an "active psychic," at a Reiki I seminar.

Ms. Strauss said that, during the Reiki II seminar, "the reiki master places symbols in the auric field to open the upper four chakras." She stated that these

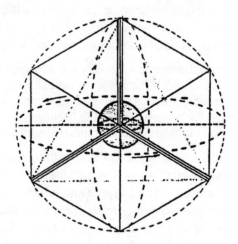

A depiction of the "antahkarana," reiki's "master frequency" symbol. The American Reiki Master Association's first-degree reiki manual states that "laying upon" it for three minutes will "reverse body magnetic poles and body polarity permanently" and thus transform one into "a channel for natural healing energies and chakra balance."

symbols can be "drawn, visualized, or blown" into the "auric field." She heartily recommended to me two books on the center's suggested reading list: *Manifesting: A Master's Manual* and Shakti Gawain's *Creative Visualization.*

Six guests and six practitioners, including reiki masters Mr. and Ms. Strauss, attended the meeting. Two of the practitioners were "reiki master candidates." One, a Japanese national who had been in the United States for about six months, told me that half of his reason for coming was to learn reiki. He said that he could have studied reiki in Japan but that it was "more powerful" here. One of the guests was a professional haircutter and former accountant from Venezuela. A flyer he gave me describes him as a "healing haircutter" and states:

> Did you know your energy comes into your body through your *head*?!?
> If you are feeling you are important on this planet and want to clean up and harmonize your energy, *then help yourself!* Call me and make your own appointment and enjoy my service.

After we introduced ourselves one by one, Mr. Strauss announced upcoming center events. Then we sang along with two recordings—"The Greatest Love of All," by George Benson, and a song titled "I Love Myself the Way I Am"—with Ms. Strauss's parakeet chirping in.

After the "sing-along," Ms. Strauss invited us to fill out absent-healing forms for our own benefit or on behalf of persons in need of "energy." She explained the use of the forms:

> In Reiki II, you learn to use symbols, and one of the symbols we use is for absentee healing—so that we can send healing to people who are not here that we're thinking of [and] who could use the energy. And what we do is, we fill it out: we put the date, the name, their age, where they're located, and what the problem is. And then we put them in the box there, and then anyone from Reiki I up can sit with the box and send healing energy this way. . . . They keep it in the box for one month.

Later, Ms. Strauss played an audiotape of instrumental New Age music and someone turned off most of the lights. Conducting a "guided meditation" session, she asked us to "visualize, sense, or touch" the number three, three times. Numbers two and one followed. She said:

> You are in that very special place where everything is perfect for you. There is no right and no wrong. This is a very special place for you and you alone. You are very protected and very loved.
> Now I'd like you to visualize a golden sphere, a round golden ball, above your head. Bring this golden ball down till it touches your crown; and, as it touches your crown, feel it opening, and feel a golden,

cleansing energy opening, relaxing, and healing. Allow this golden ball to expand there, relaxing your whole head.

Now I would like you to visualize this golden ball over your third eye; and, as this golden ball touches your third eye, feel it opening and expanding, radiating, bringing to your intuitiveness full awareness.

She further asked us to imagine the "golden sphere" at the throat chakra, "easing" our "communications"; at the heart chakra; at the stomach (solar plexus); at the pelvis; and at the base of the spine.

Afterwards, the other guests and I formed an inner circle with the practitioners outside. Behind us, they silently placed their hands on various parts of our bodies. The Strausses also touched practitioners. One practitioner had a hand on my upper back, another had a hand on my lower back, and Mr. Strauss placed his hand on the crown of my head.

One-to-one treatment followed the "healing circle." Mr. Strauss methodically touched, held, or gently manipulated various parts of my body from the top of my head to my ankles. When he was through, he filled a paper cup with water from a water cooler and asked me to drink. The other guests also received water. Ms. Strauss explained that reiki treatment precipitates "detoxification" and that drinking a large amount of water facilitates the process. One guest cried during and after her one-to-one treatment. My principal feelings were boredom and an eagerness to go home.

The next chapter deals with "psychospiritual" forms of bodywork—and more weeping.

12

Body Psychotherapy

Body-centered psychotherapy is also called body-oriented psychotherapy, body psychotherapy, direct body-contact psychotherapy, and humanistic body psychotherapy. Malcolm Brown, Ph.D., who collaborated with the founder of bioenergetics in the 1960s, describes the theoretical basis of body-centered psychotherapy in *The Healing Touch: An Introduction to Organismic Psychotherapy* (1990):

> Modern psychiatry and psychotherapy will continue to flounder in misplaced practice and irrelevant theories until they recognize the simple truth that the core of man's psyche is located not in the head, but in his total organism. The unconscious dimensions of the human psyche actually belong more to the kingdom of the body than of the mind. Furthermore, the depths and breadths of the human soul, as distinct from the mind and psyche, find their primary locus in the total organism, in its many and opposing complex fields of responsiveness.

In conventional forms of psychotherapy, little or no physical contact takes place between therapist and patient. In fact, conventional psychotherapists generally condemn such contact because it can provoke unhealthy fantasies. In contrast, all modes of body psychotherapy encourage or demand physical contact—in some cases, repeated and sustained physical contact—as a means of "unblocking" the mind. This chapter describes my sessions with two practitioners of body psychotherapy—one a "synergist," the other a "facilitator" of holotropic breathwork.

Rubenfeld Synergy

The Rubenfeld synergy method is based partly on the Alexander technique. Onetime orchestra conductor Ilana Rubenfeld developed the method in the early 1960s. A brochure describing a 1993 conference cosponsored by the Fetzer Institute (see Chapter 4) quotes her: "The body is the sacred sanctuary of the soul." According to a brochure from the Rubenfeld Center in New York City's Greenwich Village, "Emotions and memories stored in our beings often result in energy blocks, tensions, and imbalances." In a supplementary article, Rubenfeld states: "The body, mind, emotions, and spirit all form a dynamic and unitary—although not necessarily a unified—structure." Rubenfeld synergy involves aura analysis, "intentional and noninvasive" touch, kinesthesia, dreamwork, and humor. Practitioners are called "synergists."

The Rubenfeld Center referred me to Jayne Gumpel, C.S.W. (certified social worker), who directs The 36th Street Center in midtown Manhattan. I visited Ms. Gumpel there on June 9, 1993. Her fee was $90 per fifty-minute session. At the beginning of the session we sat opposite in armchairs and chatted for about four minutes. For most of the following hour, I lay on my back on a cushioned table while she touched, held, or manipulated various parts of my body. For example, she held my head in her hands, held both of my shoulders simultaneously, held both of my feet, placed her hand over mine as it rested on my chest, lifted my left arm, and poked the upper left side of my back.

Once I lay on the table, Gumpel asked me to close my eyes. She stated:

> For right now, I want to invite you to just notice how you make contact with the table. So begin by noticing the back of your head. Notice where you're most in contact with the table. And then move your awareness down to your right shoulder and shoulder blade, and notice how your right shoulder and shoulder blade contact the table.

Next, Gumpel asked me successively to turn my attention to different parts on my body's right side: arm, elbow, wrist, fingers, hip, pelvis, thigh, leg, calf, and foot. Then she asked me to "become aware of" the entire right side of my body. She inquired if I noticed any differences between my right and left sides. "Can you tell me right now what you're aware of?" she queried.

I replied that my right side seemed to be pushing more into the table than my left and that I felt as if I were inclining to the right.

"Well, let's see about that," she said. Then she repeated the foregoing procedure with the left side of my body. I concluded that my left side seemed lighter than my right.

Gumpel placed her hands on my head and neck and stated:

I'm curious about that. Are you willing to experiment with it?. . . Imagine that your left side has a voice and your right side has a voice. Can you have your left side talk to your right side? What does your left side say? Describe yourself from what you notice on the left side.

I hesitated and Gumpel said: "So tell me what you notice on the left side that's different."

"Well, I know my heart is there," I responded. "Does this mean I'm lighthearted?"

Gumpel asked me to place my left hand on my heart. "So just imagine right now that your heart has a voice," she said. "What would your heart say?"

"Relax," I answered.

"Would it say anything else?"

This question led to a shallow and useless conversation regarding career, family, and my skeptical bent. After this, Gumpel asked me to close my eyes again. She stated:

> I want to tell you that there's nothing magical about Rubenfeld synergy method, and it's not a method that's more than what happens between the two of us, you being an equal part of what happens here. So there is no magic and there is no hocus-pocus or anything special in secret that I'm doing to you. What I'm asking for is for you to move inside your body in a way that you let go of the outside and move into the inside and just notice how you live inside your body—notice your life force inside yourself, your breath.

Gumpel inquired if I noticed a "holding" or a "tension" anywhere in my body. I responded that my left shoulder felt as though it were curled upward. "So bring your awareness to your left shoulder," she said. She asked me to imagine space. "Could you tell me what image you have?"

"A broad expanse of ocean," I answered, "and a blue sky meeting it, and a white bird."

"Does that white bird have anything to say?"

"No," I responded. "Birds can't talk."

"If it could, what would it say?"

"'Give me a worm,' I suppose."

Although I was uneasy, I did not worm out of the rest of the session. Toward its end, Gumpel stated:

> What I hear you saying is that in a few ways you feel stuck. And I think the only thing that we can say about that, as far as Rubenfeld synergy method [is concerned], is that your body also responds to emotional 'stuckness.'. . . [Rubenfeld synergy] really isn't anything more pro-

found than that—even though I think it's a profound way to work, in that you 'somatize,' or your body holds onto, being stuck, just as much as your mind does. You feel the 'stuckness' in your body, 'cause you simply can't think something without also something happening. So when you think on a subtle level, you have some change in the body. Sometimes it's a gross change.... If you think you're going to be killed, what goes on in your body is pretty traumatic. If you think that you're not going to be killed but [that] you're going to be hurt, something happens. If you think that you're going ... to feel really good—like if you see an ice cream cone and you think you're going ... to eat it— something goes on in the body.

So your body responds to emotions, whether they're externally generated or internally provoked. So your body holds onto what happens to you. Your body responds to what happens to you.

That the body responds to stressors is a truism, and I so informed Ms. Gumpel. But she maintained that memories are stored in every part of the body. She explained that women who are sexually abused or raped "hold the story in their pelvis."

Holotropic Breathwork

Psychiatrist Stanislav Grof, M.D., and his wife, Christina Grof, developed holotropic breathwork in the 1970s. It involves breathing exercises, sound technology (including music), bodywork, and the drawing of mandalas—aids to meditation symbolizing the unity of the soul with the universe. One of the purported goals of holotropic therapy is to produce mystical states of awareness by releasing emotional conditions supposedly frozen in tissues. Grof claims that holotropic therapy can induce "transpersonal experiences." In *What Survives? Contemporary Explorations of Life After Death* (1990), he describes one class of these alleged results as "characterized by experiential exploration of domains that in Western culture are not considered to be part of objective reality." He further states:

> Because transpersonal experiences can convey instant intuitive information about any aspect of the universe in the present, past, and future, they appear to violate some of the most basic assumptions of mechanistic science, implying that, in a yet unexplained way, each human being contains information about the entire universe, has potential experiential access to all its parts, and in a sense *is* the whole cosmic network.

At the Breathing Art Center in Rego Park, New York, Ruth R. Klein, Ed.D., a "certified facilitator of holotropic breathwork," offers private sessions lasting three-and-a-half to five hours and group "intensives" that span about twelve hours. The private sessions cost $40 to $60 per hour and the group sessions $95 to $110 per session. On the telephone, Dr. Klein defined "holotropic" as "moving toward wholeness." She told me that holotropic breathwork may involve "focused bodywork," but that it is not an essential part of the therapy. Dr. Klein mailed me material for prospective clients, including an information sheet, a general questionnaire, and a medical questionnaire. The information sheet states:

> Holotropic breathwork is a gentle, powerful method which accesses one's natural healing energies by expanding consciousness. Developed by Dr. Stanislav Grof and Christina Grof, internationally recognized leaders in Transpersonal Psychology, this process is appropriate for those just beginning their inner journeys, as well as those already familiar with the deeper realms of the human unconscious.
>
> Facilitated by the breath, surrendering to the wisdom of body and psyche, one can contact memories, mobilize blocked feelings, heal past wounds, release barriers to our knowing our wholeness. By transforming emotional and psychosomatic symptoms into an experience of a transpersonal nature, this work offers a unique healing potential.
>
> This simple, direct approach, combining evocative music, relaxation, focused bodywork, and mandala drawing in a safe, supportive setting, honors the inner journey as sacred.

The general questionnaire addresses the client's upbringing, family history, employment, and religious background. The medical information form states that holotropic breathwork is not appropriate for persons who are pregnant, who have recently undergone surgery or a fracture, or who have cardiovascular problems, acute infectious diseases, or epilepsy.

Freelance writer Fred Levine, author of *The Psychic Sourcebook* (1988), attended a two-day holotropic therapy workshop in Boston and reported a four-hour session in the May/June 1992 issue of *East West Natural Health*:

> Ten of us lay on sleeping bags, blankets, and air mattresses around the edges of a small room, each with a companion sitting or kneeling alongside us. The lights dimmed and we were asked to close our eyes and begin breathing deeply and rapidly. "A little deeper, a little faster," a voice instructed. "A little deeper, a little faster." Suddenly, four huge speakers filled the room with the pounding of African drums. Before long, the hypnotic chants of the recording were matched by groans and wails coming from the 10 prone bodies. . . .
>
> As soon as the room exploded with the throbbing rhythms of African music, my body began a cosmic dance of its own, my arms

curling back like crab claws, my back arching upward, my legs bouncing off the ground in time with the drumming. It was all I could do to keep breathing, my face was tightly contracted into a muscle spasm, my lips frozen in a horror-mask grimace. My partner, a Harvard-trained child psychiatrist... later told me he had seen similar postures in mental wards.

My "Interrupted Journey"

On Saturday, June 19, 1993, I attended a holotropic group "intensive" at the Breathing Art Center that lasted from 8:45 A.M. to 7:45 P.M. Dr. Klein had instructed me to have a light breakfast, wear comfortable clothes, and bring a sheet and one or two pillows suitable for sleeping. Klein is a Zen Buddhist and an artist. "The universe has its reasons," she stated, "and why not trust?" She operates the center out of her home, a private house with a porch. She said she had been raised there and had returned to care for her father shortly before he died. She stated: "It's hard to be alone with all the spirits in this house." A flyer for the center describes other "opportunities for personal growth" available at the center, including "inner healing with imagery," a "chronic illness support group," and "just painting." "Just painting" is purportedly "a place to honor and relax into who we truly are, allowing creative energy to flow through us—our toes, hearts, diaphragms, fingertips—emerging in color and form."

Three other clients participated, all men apparently over thirty years old. The program consisted of a round of introductions, Klein's orientation, two breathwork periods, two artwork periods, and a "sharing session." It took place in a small living room with the blinds closed and foam cushions, pillows, and bottles of water on the parquet. During the breathwork periods, two clients lay on the cushions with their eyes closed while the other two acted as helpers—partners or "sitters." Klein said that, before each session, holotropic "breathers" and their partners should create guidelines regarding what assistance the partner will give. For example, the "breather" may ask the partner to pat him if he appears asleep, or to hold a bottle of water near his mouth whenever he touches his lips. Klein explained:

> If you need water, your partner will give you your water. If you need to use the bathroom, your partner will guide you to the bathroom. . . . If you want your partner to remind you to breathe [holotropically], you just need to let them know and give them a way to do that. . . . You might say: "Could you remind me to breathe just by breathing loudly in my ear?"

During the introduction period, Klein said her doctorate was in counseling psychology. She stated that she had met the Grofs in the 1970s and that, after training with them, she had begun conducting holotropic sessions in 1987. One participant described himself as a cabinetmaker by trade, an actor-director, and a student of yoga. Another said he was a part-time businessman and a part-time rebirther. Rebirthing, like holotropic breathwork, employs hyperventilation. Its purported goal is to resolve repressed attitudes and emotions that supposedly originated with prenatal and perinatal experiences. Practitioners encourage patients to reenact the birth process. The rebirther told us he had experienced holotropic breathwork for the first time three days before. "I feel really pretty nervous and scared," he said. The third client described himself as a musician, an inventor, and a cabdriver. He said that this session was his third with Klein.

During orientation, Klein stated:

> Once you make the choice to be here, I ask the commitment that you stay the whole day—that, no matter what comes up during the process, if you have an experience that you have to get out of here, you check with me first; and, if I agree that it's okay that you leave this room, that means that you either are in the dining room or the kitchen, or you're welcome to stay in the yard. . . . The reason is that this work facilitates non-ordinary states of consciousness and we can really go into experiencing past trauma. We can go into a non-ordinary state where our sensitivity is heightened. And, for your protection, it's important to stay for the whole day and to reach closure ["a sense of completion"].
> . . . Opening up actually is easier . . . than any of us think, but integrating—going back into the ordinary world—sometimes takes a little more doing. . . . It's very easy to kind of trip out on intense music when we're given permission, but if you're going to a scary place, how can you come to closure?. . . Part of the contract is to stay for the duration.

Klein stated that, during a session a few months before in the same room, all the participants had been sweating except one—a woman whose Arctic "experience" had left her "freezing" even with five or six blankets covering her. Klein said that some of her clients had screamed as loudly as she'd ever heard anyone scream. She expounded:

> The range is very great. . . . We can experience—and relive—childhood trauma, birth trauma. . . . and [have] experiences of past lives, future lives. We can hang out with deities. We can laugh for an hour and be in ecstasy, and we can have an experience of really being in hell and in pain. . . . What we get is really what's under the surface to come up. . . .

In this process, which is homeopathic as well as shamanic in terms of its theoretical affiliation, if somebody comes and says, "I'm feeling depressed," I'm going to say: "Allow yourself to feel completely depressed. Let go of the resistance to depression."... [If you are scared,] then allow yourself to be completely scared.

Later, she added:

You could be meeting with gods or you could be meeting with demons. You could have become a rock. You could be experiencing yourself as a tree. You could be a woman giving birth.... You could experience yourself as a victim being killed. You could be experiencing yourself as Hitler killing. I don't know what's going on, but I will assume that whatever's going on is for healing, and I will encourage you to stay with it....

There's no right or wrong.... You can't do it wrong.... There's no place to go where you're out of the ballpark. Everything's in the ballpark: having the experience, not having an experience, being with the gods, being with the ants, being happy, being unhappy.... If you have very strong sexual feelings that you want to act on, that's okay. What I will do is—to the best of my ability, which is pretty good, and with your partner's help—just afford you privacy under the covers.... Many people have had the experience of... a very, very primal connection with the earth and wanting to take clothes off.

I asked Klein if any of her clients had ever become violent. She replied:

People have expressed a great deal of violence. They have expressed it verbally and they have expressed it physically. And I'm trained to work with that. And if I need help—which I often do ... I ask for assistance from partners.... People have certainly expressed violence and rage—at life, at the cosmos, at their parents, at the church, at themselves ... at the doctor.

"The Grofs," she said, "have found that we all tend to carry one of the birth matrixes as the ground in which we live and work from." In *The Adventure of Self-Discovery* (1980), Stanislav Grof describes four "basic perinatal matrixes": (1) the "amniotic universe," (2) "cosmic engulfment and no exit," (3) the "death-rebirth struggle," and (4) the "death-rebirth experience." Klein explained: "There's like a whole constellation of experiences that surround these different stages."

She prepared us for holotropic breathing:

The breathing instructions will be to breathe faster than normal and deeper than normal. How you do that is completely individual. You can use your nose, you can use your mouth, you can do it in combination.

Your "fast" may be somebody else's "slow." Their "slow" may be your "fast." It's whatever is deeper and faster to us. There's no wrong way to do it. . . .

The music will be very loud. . . . I have earplugs if anybody really wants them. . . . If you like the music, you can go with it—great. If you can't stand it, it's part of the process. . . .

You're encouraged to stay lying down with your eyes closed the whole time. . . .

Sometimes people have an experience—because this is hyperventilating—where there's . . . a . . . spasm in [either] the hands or the feet. . . . Everything that comes up is something that is coming up to be worked through. If you have a lot of spasm and you want some massage, let me know. . . . But . . . if, let's say, your hand goes into spasm, the first thing you might want to do is to increase it, make it even worse. . . . My response to just about everything will be . . . to increase whatever your experience is. . . .

If anything feels distracting, make it part of the journey. Everything is part of the journey. . . . Sometimes people throw up. . . .

If you really feel stuck and you don't know what to do, the first thing to do is to ask for inner guidance.

The first breathwork period began shortly after ten o'clock. Klein said: "This is sacred time. If you have a connection with a god or any higher power, this is the time to make that connection." Both breathwork periods began with an instrumental melody at a restful volume, but the rest of the music was loud and often cacophonous, including chanting, sorrowful noises, and the sound of breaking glass. I developed a headache. None of the singing was in English. Later, Klein explained that facilitators try to use only songs whose lyrics are in a language their clients don't comprehend. Her audiocassette collection included "Africa Witchcraft and Ritual Music" and Sufi music for meditation.

I was a sitter during the first breathwork period. The breather under my observation, the cabbie, behaved like a restless sleeper until noon. Then, as he lay on his side, his stomach began jerking. Klein knelt beside him and placed her hand and forearm on his back. He wept. Klein whispered to him. When he lay on his stomach, she applied pressure to his back with the palm of her hand. For his mandala, the cabbie crayoned a yellow vagina with bird-wings and arthropod legs.

The other breather, the rebirther, lay like a corpse, with a sheet covering him up to his neck, until about 12:45 P.M. Then he became restless. Klein applied finger pressure to his jaws and then placed the palm of her hand over his brow. About twenty minutes later, she applied pressure to his chest with her arms and he screamed. Then he began laughing. He screamed three more times and laughed again. Klein applied finger pressure to his jaws again, while his sitter's palms lay crosswise over his forehead. He screamed again twice. "I'm having a good time!" he exclaimed. He laughed again; then he roared. Later, I asked the rebirther what had made him scream. He replied that Klein had encouraged him to "let it out" as she applied pressure to his chest.

After a lunch break, I was a breather. Breathing deeply and rapidly made me uncomfortable, so my breathing was generally natural. I was bored and eager to leave. I did not inform Klein of my boredom, perhaps fearing she might try to increase it. Hearing two familiar tunes composed by Yanni dissipated whatever absorption I had managed. Later, I told Klein I would have been more relaxed listening to such music at a lower volume alone in my study. Unlike me, the cabinetmaker huffed and puffed, then laughed or cried. "You bastard!" he roared several times. "Get away from me!" he shouted. "Don't fuck with me! Fuckin' my asshole!" (He did not appear to be speaking to anyone present.)

At about five o'clock, a burst of light made me open my eyes. Klein had opened a venetian blind. In a while, I went to the dining room to draw a mandala with crayons of various colors. A half-hour later, Klein lay embracing the cabinetmaker for about ten minutes.

During the "sharing session," he explained that his older brother had been wont to beat him up. Klein disallowed taking notes or using a tape recorder during this period. The rebirther stated he did not want to participate. He complained of a headache and uneasiness, expressed dissatisfaction with the music, and said he doubted he would continue using holotropic breathwork. He told us that during his breathwork session, he had wished he were home watching the U.S. Open golf championship. He left early. The cabdriver said he had cried in order to get his money's worth. Klein stated that my jaw looked more relaxed than it had in the morning. She said that during one breathwork session, she had witnessed the disappearance of blisters from a "breather" with poison oak dermatitis.

The Bottom Line

At best, supernaturalistic forms of bodywork promote relaxation or provide pleasant stimulation. At worst, they are painful and expensive sources of false hope. The following chapter deals with the leading source of pseudoscientific bodywork in the United States—chiropractic.

13

Mystical Chiropractic

Although some styles of chiropractic are not supernaturalistic, chiropractors have been among the chief innovators and supporters of mystical healing since the inception of their trade. Three members of my immediate family patronized chiropractors—one of whom utilized cupping—and for many years I vaguely mistook chiropractic for a branch of medicine. My preparation for this chapter included visiting a self-styled "straight mixer" and wading through some seven pounds of informational materials.

Palmer's Disjointed Legacy

Daniel David Palmer—an Iowa grocer, fish seller, spiritualist, and neo-mesmerist—devised chiropractic in 1895. Palmer postulated that the "vital force"—which he termed "Innate"—expressed itself through the nervous system. Today, some chiropractors adhere to this belief, some reject it entirely, and others occupy a nebulous middle ground in which they consider distur-bances in the flow of "nerve energy" a major or underlying cause rather than the sole cause of health problems.

Chiropractors number more than 45,000. Most can be characterized as "straights" or "mixers." "Straights" subscribe more or less to Palmer's basic doctrines that misalignments of the vertebrae—"subluxations"—cause most illnesses and that spinal "adjustments" can cure such conditions. The World Chiropractic Alliance, for example, defines straight chiropractic as "a limited, primary health care profession in which professional responsibility and author-ity are limited to the anatomy of the spine and immediate articulations [joints], the condition of vertebral subluxation, and a scope of practice which encom-

147

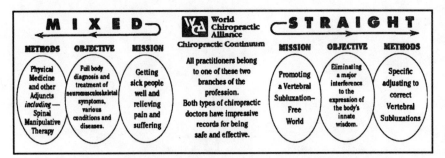

A chart used in a World Chiropractic Alliance press kit to represent the spectrum of chiropractic beliefs

passes educating, advising about, and addressing vertebral subluxations." Many straights call "subluxations" the "silent killer."

"Mixers," who outnumber straights, acknowledge the importance of germs, hormones, and other factors in disease but tend to regard mechanical disturbances of the nervous system as a fundamental cause. Besides spinal manipulation, mixers may employ nutritional supplementation, homeopathic "remedies," acupressure, enemas, and various forms of physiotherapy (heat, cold, traction, exercise, massage, and ultrasound).

A third category of chiropractors comprises only a few hundred who reject Palmer's philosophy and have pledged to restrict treatment to "neuromusculoskeletal conditions of a nonsurgical nature." Their apparent aim is to convert chiropractors into scientific physical therapists without loss of the title "doctor." In the May 1992 issue of *Chiropractic Technique*, reformer Samuel Homola, D.C., states:

> I am distressed by the propaganda of chiropractic organizations that use back pain studies to promote the chiropractor as a "family physician."
> While it appears that chiropractors might have the best treatment for mechanical-type back trouble, few chiropractors claim to be back specialists. Most chiropractors present themselves as "general practitioners" who offer treatment for a variety of health problems. . . .
> After 35 years of practice as a chiropractor, I have not been convinced that slightly misaligned vertebrae can be harmful to health.

A recent flyer from the International Chiropractors Association titled "11 Common Questions about Chiropractic" states that, even if one feels fine, chiropractic "care" is advisable for maintenance of a required level of health and fitness, that periodic "adjustments" can increase resistance to disease and may be necessary for health maintenance, and that chiropractic treatment is appropriate for persons of all ages. Further, it suggests that chiropractic is the best "first response" to most illnesses and injuries. Such claims are the stock-in-trade of chiropractors, many of whom routinely recommend weekly or monthly "adjustments" throughout life.

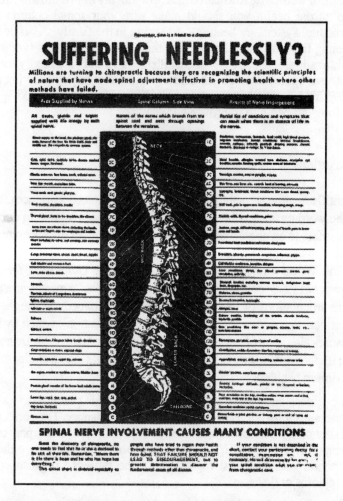

This "spine chart," sold by a prominent chiropractic equipment and supply house, lists more than a hundred symptoms and conditions that supposedly result from "nerve impingement." The conditions include appendicitis, crossed eyes, diabetes, high and low blood pressure, and hardening of the arteries. During the 1970s, the company's catalog described the chart as "an inexpensive way to enhance patient indoctrination programs and answer patient questions."

In 1991, Ted Koren, D.C., published the flyer "Why Should I Go to a Chiropractor?," which states:

> Feeling "good" is not the same as being healthy. Too many people who felt "good" have been told they had silent cancers growing within them, or were close to a heart attack, or suddenly fell victim to a stroke! To ensure health you should make sure your spinal column and structural system are healthy—and bring in the family! . . . If you're feeling fine you should remember that spinal nerve stress (vertebral subluxations) are painless "silent killers." You and your family should get your spines checked periodically to make sure you're living free from hidden spinal nerve stress. . . . Why wait for disease to happen before you begin to improve your health?

"Subluxations"

In scientific healthcare, subluxations are unambiguous occurrences. In medicine, the word means partial displacement of a bone in a joint. In dentistry, it usually refers to an abnormal loosening of teeth without displacement. However, the typical chiropractic "subluxation" is imaginary.

The World Chiropractic Alliance's *Practice Guidelines for Straight Chiropractic* (1993) defines "vertebral subluxation" as "a misalignment of one or more articulations of the spinal column or its immediate weight-bearing articulations, to a degree less than a luxation [dislocation], which by interference causes alteration of nerve function and interference to the transmission of mental impulses, resulting in a lessening of the body's innate ability to express its maximum health potential." It further states:

> The professional practice objective of straight chiropractic is to correct vertebral subluxations in a safe and effective manner. The correction of subluxations is not considered to be a specific cure for any particular symptom or disease. It is applicable to any patient who exhibits vertebral subluxation(s) regardless of the presence or absence of symptoms or disease.

The nature of the chiropractic subluxation is slippery, even to many chiropractors. While some chiropractors depict subluxations as "bones out of place," others describe them quite vaguely. The December 1986 issue of the *Journal of Chiropractic* includes a perspective by Vincent P. Lucido, D.C., titled "The Dilemma of 'Subluxation.'" Lucido, who later became president of the American Chiropractic Association, stated: "There is no consistent, widely accepted definition of subluxation within the profession." He offered *six*

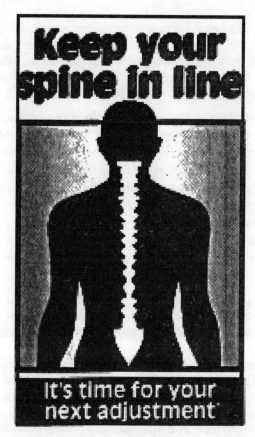

Keep your spine in line

It's time for your next adjustment

A card used to remind patients about appointments

definitions. One describes subluxation as "a complex biomechanical neuro-physiological disrelationship" that predominantly affects the spine and is usually not structural—that is, not demonstrable with an x-ray photograph.

According to the ninth edition of *Introduction to Chiropractic: A Natural Method of Health Care* (1988), chiropractic's premise is that "many ills come about as a result of improper (too much or too little) nerve supply." This "patient education" book says that chiropractors endeavor to restore proper nerve function by "adjusting" vertebrae—usually by hand—in areas that exhibit "derangements (subluxations)." The author, Louis Sportelli, D.C., is a former board chairman of the American Chiropractic Association.

In the September 1988 *American Journal of Chiropractic Medicine*, Joseph C. Keating, Jr., Ph.D., a research professor at a chiropractic college, stated:

Subluxation has become a holy word in chiropractic. Chiropractors, although unable to reach consensus on its definition and clinical significance, by and large accept that subluxations are real, that they can be detected, adjusted (reduced or eliminated), and that the patient's health will improve as a consequence.

Because subluxation theory wanders far from knowledge of human physiology, the scientific community has long rejected it. In 1968, for example, the U.S. Department of Health, Education, and Welfare concluded in a major study: "There is no valid evidence that subluxation, if it exists, is a significant factor in disease processes. Therefore, the broad application to health care of a diagnostic procedure such as spinal analysis and a treatment procedure such as spinal adjustment is not justified."

A few years later, Yale anatomy professor Edmund S. Crelin, Ph.D., D.Sc., physically demonstrated that chiropractic "subluxations" do not occur. In *Examining Holistic Medicine* (1985), he recounted his classic experiment:

I dissected out the intact spines or vertebral columns, with their attached ligaments, from three infants and three adults a few hours after they died. I carefully exposed the spinal nerves as they pass through the intervertebral openings or foramina. I placed the spines in an ordinary drill press. A fine wire was then wrapped around the spinal nerve and another was placed against the side wall of the intervertebral foramen. I then applied a measured force to both the front and back of each vertebra. I also twisted and bent the spines with a measured force. If the intervertebral foramen became reduced in size to the point that its walls merely touched the spinal nerve passing through it, the wires would also touch and cause a volt-ohm-microampere meter to register it. The forces applied to the spine reached the level where the spine was about to break. In not one instance did the walls of the intervertebral foramina impinge on the nerves passing through them. In order to have that happen I had to break the spine.

Dr. Crelin added that spinal pressure on nerves is *less* probable in living bodies because of the counteractive response of powerful spinal muscles.

Despite such findings, Palmer's theory appears entrenched in state and federal laws. Medicare authorizes payment for the treatment of "subluxations demonstrated by x-rays to exist," and many states license chiropractors to treat subluxations, free impinged nerves, and remove "interference" with the "transmission" or "expression" of "nerve energy" or "nerve force." For example, North Carolina law defines chiropractic as "the science of adjusting the cause of disease by realigning the spine, releasing pressure on nerves radiating from the spine to all parts of the body, and allowing the nerves to carry their full quota of health current (nerve energy) from the brain to all parts of the body." South Dakota law permits chiropractors to perform "meridian therapy" but does not define such treatment.

The Unbearable Lightness of "Innate"

In *The Chiropractic Story* (1968), Marcus Bach, Ph.D., an acquaintance of Palmer's son "B.J.," defined "Innate" as "the focus of divine mind expressed through mortal mind, challenging the latter to recognize its essence as divine." He posited two forms of "Innate": "personalized" and "corporate" (collective). Bach wrote:

> Science is the servant, Innate the executive. This is as true collectively as it is individually and as the corporate Innate grows in and through chiropractic, so grows the power of its healing force. . . .
>
> Something in the human body wishes and wills . . . to be well and stay well. Chiropractic believes that nerves send the life-force to every muscle and tissue, sustaining every organ, flowing through every impulse, attending every action, governing every thought. The nexus through which this power flows is the spine. The coil of life is in the spine. . . .
>
> Every religion no less than every spiritually-oriented approach to health and healing believes in the existence of this life force. Call it Consciousness. Call it Innate. Call it God. There is a *power* particularized in man and its most dynamic expression is *health*.

In his first book, D.D. Palmer claimed: "Too much or not enough nerve energy is disease." It would be reasonable for uninitiated laypersons to surmise that such ideas lie at the bottom of chiropractic's philosophical dustbin. However, in the Summer 1992 issue of *Philosophical Constructs for the Chiropractic Profession*, Joseph H. Donahue, D.C., states that the concept of "Innate" may be gaining acceptance among chiropractors and that possibly as many as 80 percent subscribe to some version of it. He ascribes seven traditional principles regarding the notion to a chiropractic textbook published in 1927. These hold that "Innate": (1) is the source of all material qualities and actions, (2) unites with matter to create life, (3) is inborn, (4) has the "mission" of maintaining life, (5) adapts "universal forces" and matter to the needs of the body, (6) counteracts "universal forces," and (7) operates through the nervous system in animal organisms. Donahue writes that D.D. Palmer regarded innate intelligence as a segment of "universal intelligence." In a cogent article, he opines that it is a harmful belief and concludes:

Since the concept of II [innate intelligence] is both untestable and falsified by everyday experience, it has no place in a scientific healing profession's philosophizing. . . . The uncritical world view fostered by II is held together with the glue of rationalism and evasions. The doctor, claiming to only be a "channel" for II, can evade professional accountability. The trick to evading accountability, and yet keeping the patients coming, is to imply a lot of benefits without saying anything specific. . . . .Patients can . . . be strung along with assurances that the chiropractor is doing everything possible to release the patient's II.

A flyer titled "The Force Is Within You," published in 1990 by practice-building consultant Dennis P. Nitikow, D.C., distinguishes "innate intelligence" from "life force":

There is an innate intelligence within each of us that is far superior to our educated brain which creates and recreates us on a continual basis. In order for this process to occur, life force (mental impulse) must be flowing throughout the body to all cells and tissues. . . . The innate intelligence directs this life force to every cell and tissue of the body. When the life force is free of interference the body is at its maximum health potential. If the life force is interfered with the body does not have the ability to recreate itself normally and disease results. . . .
    The Chiropractor's job is to remove the subluxation allowing the mental impulse to get to the tissue cells and replace the abnormal cells with normal cells. This is healing.

The 1993 Koren flyer "Why Should I Go to a Chiropractor?" states:

To some people, chiropractic is something strange or mysterious. . . . The goal of the doctor of chiropractic is to turn on your inner doctor, your own natural healing ability, by correcting spinal nerve stress (vertebral subluxations), one of the deadliest, most destructive blockages of life and energy that we can suffer from. This promotes natural healing, vitality, strength and health.

In 1981, reporter Mark Brown consulted, as a patient, about two dozen chiropractors in or near Davenport, Iowa, the birthplace of the trade. The December 13, 1981 issue of *Quad-City Times* carried his exhaustive investigative report, which stated: "To many chiropractors, Innate is an almost mystical presence—'the power of God being expressed in the body.'. . . Others seem to suggest that Innate is God." One chiropractor told Brown that his ears protruded because they were "antennae" for "nerve energy" and claimed that this "energy" flows through the body and out of the mouth. One morning, Brown visited a chiropractor and "learned" that his right leg was shorter than his left. Later that day, another chiropractor came to the reverse conclusion.

Brown saw chiropractor Harlow Wells in response to an ad for a free spinal exam. During his second visit to Wells, he lay on his back on a table and held up his arm at the chiropractor's request. Brown described this visit in his report:

According to the procedure, Wells would try to pull down my arm. I would resist. Under normal circumstances, my arm would remain strong. But by Wells' pressing or poking different spots on my body, the arm would give way, I had learned. He told me that muscle weakness corresponded to other health problems.

Wells tested the arm. It remained strong. Then he reached for the potato [he had brought from another room] and placed it on my chest. WHAMMO! When he pulled, my arm dropped like a rock.

"I guess this means I shouldn't put any potatoes on my chest?" Brown ventured. The chiropractor replied that potatoes would have the same effect regardless of their position on the body. He performed the same procedure with an egg and explained that enzymes and other constituents of the potato and the egg had acted unfavorably on the reporter's "aura." Wells claimed that this "interference" indicated a health problem—probably a nutritional deficiency. After further "testing" of the same sort, he sold four bottles of "glandular" supplements to Brown for $47.50.

In the first (1993) issue of the *Journal of Chiropractic Humanities*, Craig Nelson, D.C., a faculty member at Northwestern College of Chiropractic, states:

The various chiropractic techniques, in addition to prescribing corrective procedures, usually come complete with a theoretical framework to explain the rationale behind the technique. Explicitly or implicitly, each of these techniques claims a unique relationship with the truth. . . . There is no comparable circumstance in any other health profession.

B.E.S.T.—or Worst?

The Morter HealthSystem—whose purported mission is "to improve the health of mankind worldwide"—melds subluxation theory with other esoterica. The system includes B.E.S.T. (bio energetic synchronization technique), baby B.E.S.T., a stress-management program called "The Twelve Steps to Stress Less," and nutritional supplementation "to restore the body to its natural alkaline state." B.E.S.T., the centerpiece of the system, is a pseudonatural variant of self-healing and polarity balancing (see Chapter 12). M.T. Morter, Jr.,

M.A., D.C., past-president of two chiropractic colleges, developed the method in 1974 and describes it as an "approach to non-forceful chiropractic." In *B.E.S.T.* (1980), he claims that an "internal force"—"Innate Intelligence"—totally regulates health, that "Nature" is "not only smarter than we think" but "smarter than we *can* think," and that the body "does not know how to be sick."

In a booklet titled *Baby B.E.S.T.: Infant Adjusting/Care* (1991), Morter states:

> The human body was obviously built utilizing subconscious information, as neither our own nor our mother's consciousness was necessary for the nine months our body was in development. This subconsciousness in man could be thought of as a derivative of the perfect God consciousness that created us. Both GOD consciousness and the consciousness that built us are beyond the comprehension of man. Unlike some would have us believe, God is neither limited by, nor is a reflection of, the subconsciousness of man. The Universal Intelligence, or God, is much more than man can even perceive.

An introductory Morter videotape titled "The Health Revolution: Re-Inventing Healthcare" declares: "By applying today's scientific knowledge to the doctrines of yesterday, we will create the healing science of the twenty-first century." It conveys D.D. Palmer's claims that "innate intelligence" has "the power to conceive, judge and reason on matters which pertain to the internal welfare of the body" and that "the determining causes of disease are traumatism, poison and auto-suggestion." According to the videotape, trauma, toxicity, and thoughts produce "memory-retained engrams" (physical changes in nervous tissue) that interfere with sensory nerves. Such interference allegedly causes "subluxations." The narrator explains: "Bioenergy—the electromagnetic energy of the universal intelligence that creates and sustains all life—flows through the nervous system naturally. But when negative memory engrams interfere with normal bioenergy, disease happens." A 1992 videotape cites Kirlian photography.

One of the main premises of B.E.S.T. is that even weak magnetic fields have substantial effects on muscular strength. In *Baby B.E.S.T.*, Morter claims that an electromagnetic field controls the development and repair of the body throughout life. He further claims that physical trauma, chemical stresses (primarily nutritional), and mental stresses affect the movement of this field and may appear as vertebral subluxations, organic disease, or emotional disorders. B.E.S.T. supposedly "neutralizes" impediments to the electromagnetic field. Treatment involves applying finger-pressure to equally tender "pulsating points" on the body until—and for at least twenty seconds after—their pulsations synchronize. B.E.S.T. distinguishes between north and south contact-points and between "north-contact" and "south-contact" fingers. It localizes north contact-points on the half of the body that is farther from the earth—regardless of the body's position—and south contact-points on the other half. North-contact fingers are the right middle finger and the left index finger. South-contact fingers are the left middle finger and the right index finger. According to B.E.S.T., practitioners must use north-contact fingers on north contact-points and south-contact fingers on south contact-points.

Baby B.E.S.T. is an adaptation of B.E.S.T. to infants. In *Baby B.E.S.T.*, Morter states that the main objective of this variant is "the removal of segmentation imbalances to restore symmetry to the child." This allegedly "allows for an updating of the neurological responses to and from the brain." In *B.E.S.T.*, he claims that the left leg of acutely ill infants is usually shorter than the right, and that this "configuration" indicates "reversed polarity." The Morter HealthSystem *Level II Child Care & Adjusting* videotape purports to demonstrate that balancing the flow of electromagnetic energy results in instantaneous equalization of leg length.

Just Between Us "Innates"...

Concept therapy is a pseudonatural chiropractic system based on the notion of "Innate to Innate communication." The system's originator, chiropractor Thurman Fleet (1895–1983), introduced it in 1931, and his son, George T. Fleet, Jr., promotes it through the Concept-Therapy Institute, in San Antonio, Texas. An institute flyer states: "The Human is a *soul* (psyche), and has what he or she calls a *mind* and a *body*." Concept therapy comprises a "diagnostic" phase— zone therapy diagnosis—and a "therapeutic" phase—suggestive therapy.

Chiropractor Eddie Harrison described the "diagnostic" phase in the November 1990 issue of *The American Chiropractor*:

> It divides the nervous system and body into six Health Zones: Glandular, Eliminative, Nerve, Digestive, Muscular, [and] Circulatory Zones. There are six corresponding reflex points on each side of the occiput [back of the head] and four vertebrae associated with each Health Zone. Analysis consists of locating the most sensitive point on the occiput, indicating which Zone is stressed, and then specific adjustments are given to the subluxated vertebrae. If the adjustment is correct, there is an immediate reduction of tenderness on the reflex point. This is very impressive to the new patient. Zone testing at lay lectures is a winning procedure. People love it.

Suggestive therapy, the "therapeutic" phase of concept therapy, involves spinal "adjustments," "healing suggestions," a diet "to eliminate toxins,"

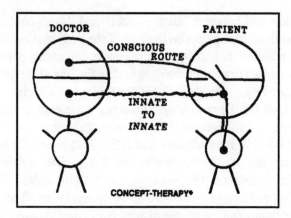

Diagram from Concept-Therapy Institute flyer

and food combining. The basis of suggestive therapy is D.D. Palmer's interpretation of autosuggestion. In scientific medicine, the term "autosuggestion" refers to the process whereby individuals accept an idea or plan and then adjust their behavior to it. For example, a smoker may convince himself that smoking entails an inordinate risk and *thereby* quit. Palmer, however, apparently regarded autosuggestion both as a key cause of disease and as a variant of self-healing. In *Text-Book of the Science, Art and Philosophy of Chiropractic for Students and Practitioners* (1910), he wrote:

> In auto-suggestion, which is also known as psychological suggestion and traumatic suggestion, the will and judgment are more or less suppressed and auto-traumatic action is directed to any organ or portion of the body, thereby modifying bodily functions, exciting or relieving morbid conditions by mental processes independently of external influence.

In a booklet titled *The Cause of Disease* (1967), Thurman Fleet expounded:

> Intense thinking about disease is probably what Dr. Palmer meant by *autosuggestion*. Intense thinking about a disease or ailment will, in time, create the disease in the body. . . . A person can center his mind on some *negative aspect of health*, or disease, and actually [create] a thing in his mind called a concept. A concept is a group of ideas put together, with precision, which becomes a thing—either a *bad thing* for the body or a *good thing*. . . .
> People use their *thinking power* to think negatively and thereby bring upon themselves deplorable conditions. This power can be used for good or evil, for health or disease. . . .

A person suffering from a functional disease, or disorder, must go to the doctor in whom he or she has faith. Faith is the *key* that opens the door to the *Innate Healing Power.* . . . .
When a doctor, seeking a cure, goes to. . . people [who teach any technique] and becomes *sold* on what they teach him, he goes back to his office and, with faith in that system, he explains it to his patient and transfers his faith over to him or her. Then the patient gets well by that particular system.

Accordingly, a Concept-Therapy Institute flyer claims that concept therapy enables doctors to cure "under any and all systems." A circular for a 1992 seminar claimed:

How you deliver your adjustment to reduce subluxations carries with it a vibratory suggestion that directs the Innate Intelligence to speed up or delay the patient's recovery. . . .
The doctor's thoughts, ideas, and inner feelings are transmitted to the patient vibratorily. The doctor who learns the hook-up between Doctor Innate and Patient Innate becomes a powerful broadcaster of health and success. Herein lies the discovery of getting patients well and attracting a bigger practice.

In a booklet titled *Suggestive Therapy Applied: The Chiropractic Approach to the Treatment of Psychosomatic Disorders* (1977), Thurman Fleet wrote:

If the Doctor holds in his mind a picture of what he wants that [patient's] body to do and be, he will then give the instructions to the Innate of that body as to what it is to do. If that person has perfect faith in the Doctor, the *composite personality* has been established—the two have become one in healing—then the mind of that patient, his conscious mind, accepts your image and your adjustment, and immediately the "trapdoor" to the Innate is opened. That image which you have given, along with the physical adjustment, activates the Innate Intelligence within the patient so that it will manifest exactly what you desire it to do.

An institute flyer illustrates the relationship between the "diagnostic" and "therapeutic" phases of concept therapy:

Improper eating habits cause. . . [the digestive] zone to be out of order in the majority of cases and it is most often in a state of subluxation. With Suggestive Therapy the Doctor, through the Chiropractic adjustment and proper suggestion, can impress the Innate Mind of the patient with the concept of perfect digestive health and the expression of health will result in the patient's body. . . .

In treating circulatory disorders which may be functional, there is more involved than merely moving a bone. The Doctor, having diagnosed the cause, must create an image to accompany the adjustment. Then ... this image of Perfect Circulatory Health is transferred to the Innate Mind of the patient which will begin the expression of bodily health.

Concept therapy is thus a "winning" combination of fundamentalist chiropractic, creative visualization, faith healing, food combining, psychic healing, and self-healing. If this isn't religion, what is?

My First Chiropractic Exam

Chiropractor John Crescione and a colleague operate the BQE Chiropractic Wellness Center in Woodside, New York. Their facility occupies a narrow "suite" inside a health spa called the BQE Racquetball and Fitness Center, of which I have been a member. An information sheet from Crescione's office states that he has a B.S. degree in nutrition and a strong background in exercise physiology. Over several years, I have collected flyers from the office that include the following assertions:

- Food preservatives and additives add considerable stress to the body. ... And anything which affects body chemistry could also affect the muscles which keep the spine in balance, thereby causing subluxation.

- The death of a loved one, separation from a spouse or any other emotionally-charged trauma often creates physical difficulties. ... Pain will occur where it never did before. This is often the sign of an emotionally-induced subluxation.

- A chiropractic spinal adjustment is one of the best things that could happen to a child (or adult) suffering from ear infection.

- If drugs truly corrected health problems, then they would only have to be taken once. ... Drugs lie to you.

- Tiredness, fatigue and exhaustion are one of the early signs of vertebral subluxations.

- Healing is indeed one of nature's miracles. It is as miraculous and mysterious as the miracle of birth.

One of the flyers states that a chiropractic examination is "essential" if a child has asthma, bronchitis, colic, constipation, a cough, a sore throat, frequent colds, a sinus problem, a fever, an ear infection, a hearing impairment, an eye problem, hypertension, numbness, poor posture, scoliosis, a skin disorder, or a pain in the arm, hand, leg, foot, head, neck, shoulder, hip, stomach, or a joint.

During the summer of 1993, a sign in the window of the BQE Chiropractic Wellness Center offered a free spinal exam and consultation. I made an appointment for August 10. Shortly after my arrival, the receptionist asked me to complete a case-history form that included the question, "How long has it been since you really felt good?" As I did so, the chiropractor gave dietary advice to a trim passerby he knew:

> It's not what you're eating [that's important]; it's the quantity. If you're working out heavy, there needs to be a constant supply of nutrition in the body so that your cells...will be able to constantly give you nutrition for healing and growth. It's not having two other meals somewhere in the course of your day [that's important]; there has to be a meal—not a full-course meal, because you won't be able to sit down and eat five times a day, but enough of a meal where you're getting enough protein, carbs, and, you know, blah, blah, blah. All right. Now, that's the dietary change you make. Get used to eating more, so that you have more fuel.
> . . . [Telling you] to eat this but not eat this and eat this [is] too complicated. Right now, get used to eating food. I'm a simple man.

The acquaintance thanked him.

I informed Crescione that I was a health writer who had never consulted a chiropractor and that this inexperience had motivated me to see him. "Oh, boy!" he responded. "You picked the right guy to come to." He briefly described his credentials and said his wife was a registered dietitian. He stated that he'd elected not to pursue a career in exercise physiology because he'd gotten tired of administering tests. "You can call me John," he said. "I'm pretty laid-back."

I had indicated low-back pain as my major complaint on the case-history form but told Crescione that I had not had it recently. As I lay fully clothed on my back on a slender table, he asked me to counteract pressure from his hand with one, and then the other, of my variously outstretched arms. With his other hand, he poked different parts of my body. He explained: "All I'm doing right now is trying to ascertain the muscle strength and position of the pelvis in relation to your muscle strength, in relation to your entire nervous system. The tests may be similar [to those of physical therapy], but the reason that we're doing them is different." With my arms relaxed, he continued poking, evidently searching for tenderness.

He asked me if I tended to yawn in the afternoon, and I said I did. Then I lay on my stomach. He began poking me alternately on the left and right sides of my body and asking me which side was more sensitive. Next, he initiated a procedure involving my legs that was similar to his previous "tests" of arm strength.

Crescione's primitive tests contrast acutely with the precise, high-tech evaluative procedures familiar to certified athletic trainers, exercise physiologists, and registered physical therapists. Yet he stated that his procedure was "more complicated" than that of many chiropractors because he was "more thorough." He expounded:

> You have a lot of chiropractors who are fairly simple and straightforward: if it hurts here, that's where you adjust it. With me, if it hurts here, yes, the problem may be here, but let's just see if it's here or if it's coming from someplace else: because, if it's here, [it's] easy [to correct]; if it's coming from someplace else and I just adjust here because you say it hurts, I'm going to create another problem. And I'm not going to do that.
>
> To really take care of somebody, chiropractically, do it right. It's actually a very specific science. . . .
>
> What chiropractic really is doing is trying to help keep the nervous system free and clear. So the spine. . . is where you start from. But [as] muscles move bones, you have to worry about the muscles: Are they too strong or too weak or what?
>
> If you're feeding nutrition into the body. . . that nutrition breaks down and it goes into muscles, tendons, and ligaments. If you're putting junk into the system, you're putting junk into tendons and ligaments and muscles.

"So I gather you're a mixer," I said.

"You're probably better off calling me a straight mixer," Crescione responded.

He claimed he had detected neurological "weaknesses." When I asked if he attributed them to backbone pressure on my nerves, he replied: "Yes. Some of it's [by the] spinal bone; some of it's by soft tissue."

When I asked Crescione whether he performed cranial balancing, he said it was a must. He concluded that I had a sprained sacroiliac joint and was "falling apart." He stated that I should resume weightlifting to prevent low-back pain— even though I had told him that the symptom had disappeared after I'd quit weightlifting. He added that the (alleged) sacroiliac-joint sprain was causing digestive problems involving the pancreas. He told me:

> The mid-thoracic area is one of the places that supply the pancreas. So if you get stuck ["subluxated"] in the mid-thoracic area, you get a change in nerve flow from that nerve out to the pancreas. So what does

the pancreas do? Sugar metabolism. That's your energy. So a lot of those afternoon yawns may be coming from that thoracic [area] being stuck.

He advised me to get an x-ray, for $50, at his other office.

The chiropractor enumerated my options: (1) I could do nothing; (2) I could seek a second opinion from a physical therapist or exercise physiologist; (3) I could submit to chiropractic treatment of "spinal misalignments or spinal subluxations"; or (4) I could avail myself of his counseling services concerning nutrition and exercise "to get as much change into the nervous system as possible." However, he warned me: "I'll tell you now: this low-back pain . . . will recur again, and it will get progressively worse to the point where you're not going to be able to get up, and then you'll be out."

"But it hasn't gotten worse," I countered.

"It will," he asserted. "You may not have a big problem there until you're in your forties or fifties [I was 39], and then it's going to come in a form of a disc that they want to take out. That's your choice."

When I inquired about fees, Crescione said I needed dietary counseling, spinal "adjusting," and possibly applied kinesiology—"the icing on the cake"— just to treat *one* of my "different problems": my tendency to yawn in the afternoon, which he termed a "digestive thing." He estimated that at least two sessions per week for six to twelve weeks would be sufficient to correct these problems. The quoted cost per session was $40.

Not long after my visit, Crescione's office made expiration-dated "certificates" available elsewhere in the health spa entitling bearers to a free exam. I also overheard an employee of the health spa tell a potential member: "When you join, you can get a free spinal analysis."

Chiropractic's Bottom Line

National Council Against Health Fraud president William T. Jarvis, Ph.D., has noted that physiotherapists, athletic trainers, and various medical specialists sometimes use manipulation to treat certain musculoskeletal problems. Jarvis explains:

> Chiropractic's uniqueness lies not in its use of manipulation but in its theoretical basis for doing so—which also explains why chiropractors overutilize spinal manipulation, often applying it without justification. The fact that most of their schools are accredited reflects the failure of the U.S. Office of Education to require that health professions whose accrediting agencies they recognize be scientifically valid.

In the July 1991 issue of *Philosophical Constructs for the Chiropractic Profession*, William Bachop, Ph.D., professor of anatomy at National College of Chiropractic, provided a sobering critique of chiropractic's theoretical basis. In an article titled "The Warfare of Science with Philosophy in Contemporary Chiropractic," Bachop stated:

> What is called "Chiropractic Philosophy" turns out to be a creed, and what is pointed to as philosophical discourse is more like a sermon preached to the converted. . . .
> The defenders of the chiropractic faith are not true philosophers: they are true believers. They denounce change as apostasy. They call upon the faithful to resist heresy. The principal heresy is any science that flies in the face of their doctrines or, better said, dogmas. When science happens to agree with some doctrine of theirs, no one is allowed to forget that science is in agreement with them. But when science disagrees, one is sanctimoniously told that science is a limited way of knowing and that chiropractic philosophy is a way of knowing that transcends the limitations of science. . . . So science becomes a buffet from which one selects those scientific tidbits that satisfy one's taste.

These comments are germane to other forms of "alternative" healthcare.

Some Final Thoughts about "Alternative" Healthcare

In the nineteenth century, when many fringe "healing" systems became popular, orthodox medicine was largely unfounded. Today, however, scientific medicine is based on a coherent body of reproducible experiments.

Practitioners of "alternative" healthcare do not conform to current scientific standards. Instead, they variously—and often seductively—cater to desires for attention, for a sounding board, for participatory entertainment, desires to feel understood, to be touched and held without threat, and to be treated as more than cut-and-dried matter. However, the price of such emotional gratification may include deadly confusion about health, disease, and healing.

I believe that the best defense against—and antidote for—mystical thinking and the health-related claims that nourish it is a humane and thoroughly secular education that emphasizes science and reasonable, constructive skepticism. Once it takes hold, skepticism has a tremendous scope and a tendency to proliferate. Therein lies its promise—and an advantage I lacked throughout some twenty-two years of academic enrollment.

Glossary of
Supernaturalistic Methods

Absent healing (distant healing, distance healing, remote healing, absentee healing, teleotherapeutics): Alleged treatment of a patient, who is not in the practitioner's vicinity, through magic, meditation, prayer, "spirit doctors," or telepathy. According to *The Concise Lexicon of the Occult* (1990), absent healing is "a form of faith healing involving the projection of positive healing energy."

Actualism (agni yoga, fire yoga, lightwork): Modern offshoot of yoga whose goals, according to the New York Actualism Center, are the integration of body, mind, identity, and spirit and "the awakening to and empowerment of the goodness, beauty and truth of YOU." (See Chapter 5.)

Actualism bodywork: System of massage "designed to help awaken the body and its consciousness to the indwelling Creator, and to the Creator's love," according to the New York Actualism Center. The system includes fourteen basic bodywork patterns and four combination patterns. The center defines each pattern in terms of anatomy and purported utility. The pattern designated "foot," for example, supposedly leaves the client's feet "feeling happy and appreciated," enhances the ability to breathe, and "opens" the feet to facilitate "unloading" of the entire body. "Nerve work" allegedly helps extend the client's sensory awareness and deepen enjoyment of "life-energies."

Acu-ball pressure self-treatment: Form of self-applied acupressure characterized by the use of soft, solid-rubber balls.

Acupressure (*G-jo*): Any treatment involving the stimulation of acupuncture points either with the hands alone or with hand-held tools. "Acupressure" may also refer specifically to shiatsu (see below). *G-jo* is Chinese for "first aid."

Acupuncture (acupuncture therapy): Insertion of needles of various shapes into the skin to stimulate hypothetical "acupoints." Practitioners sometimes insert the needles parallel to the body surface. At other times, they insert the needles to the depth of the periosteum (the membrane covering the bones)—a method called periosteal acupuncture. Acupuncture is supposedly based on "unknown laws." Practitioners also stimulate acupoints with electricity, lasers, and ultrasound. (See Chapters 3 and 4.)

Acuscope therapy (electro-acuscope therapy): Computerized system that supposedly enables assessment and treatment of virtually any injury. The "acuscope" is a device that allegedly normalizes acupuncture points by means of a weak electric current.

Acu-yoga: Combination of self-applied acupressure and a set of yogic postures and stretches. Acu-yoga supposedly activates the "acupoints" and "energy pathways" of acupuncture. Proponents recommend it for menstrual irregularity and premenstrual tension syndrome (PMS) and to strengthen the immune system.

African holistic health: Ethnic variant of naturopathy (see Chapter 8) forged by certified herbalist and massage therapist Dr. Llaila O. Afrika. The February/March 1991 issue of *Upscale* quotes him: "European medicine—the use of synthetic drugs and surgery—is organized to treat symptoms. African medicine is organized to treat the physical, mental and spiritual causes of dis-ease."

Agni dhatu (*agni dhatu* **therapy,** *samadhi* **yoga):** Spiritual mode of bodywork that purportedly tranquilizes the subconscious and causes "core tissues" to "bloom."

Aikido: Spiritual discipline and self-defense method that employs grappling, throws, and "nonresistance" to debilitate opponents. "Aikido" combines three terms: *ai* ("union" or "harmony"), *ki* ("breath," "spirit," or "life force"), and *do* ("way"). Proponents translate "aikido" as "the way of unifying *ki*" or "the way of harmony with the spirit of the universe (or universal energy)." Morihei Ueshiba (1883–1969), a Japanese farmer and master martial artist, founded aikido sometime between 1922 and 1931—supposedly after a divine revelation. Ueshiba claimed he possessed supernatural power. (His surname is also spelled "Oyeshiba" and "Uyeshiba.") In *Japan: Strategy of the Unseen* (1987), Michel Random wrote: "In *aikido*, the secret is to make a void, directing it either against the adversary, who thus finds himself as it were enclosed in a circle from which he cannot escape, or drawing him into the void of one's own circle." Practitioners sometimes promote aikido as a vitalistic "health practice."

Alchemical hypnotherapy (alchemical work): Form of hypnotism developed by David Quigley. The Alchemical Hypnotherapy Institute, in Santa Rosa, California, describes alchemical hypnotherapy as a synthesis of techniques and concepts from Jungian and transpersonal psychology, neurolinguistic programming, past-life therapy, psychosynthesis, and shamanism (see below for all). It is allegedly designed "to assist the client in working with their Inner Guides to change their lives."

Alexander technique (Alexander method): Murky "body/mind" method focused on posture improvement. Maintaining alignment of the head, neck, and back supposedly leads to optimum overall physical functioning. Proponents claim that the technique is useful in treating a variety of diseases, including asthma, hypertension, peptic ulcer disease, and ulcerative colitis. Frederick Matthias Alexander (1869–1955), an Australian Shakespearean actor, developed the method at the turn of the century. Although his original purpose was to assist voice projection, Alexander concluded that faulty posture was responsible for diverse symptoms. He postulated that habitual unbalanced movement affects the functioning of the entire body—implying that postures entail behavior patterns and that bad postural habits can distort one's personality. Alexander further postulated that all proper bodily movements flowed from one basic movement—the maximum lengthening of the spine—which he termed the "primary control." Teachers convey the technique by manually applying gentle pressure to various parts of the student's body and simultaneously repeating key phrases. (See Chapter 11.)

Alternative twelve steps: Nontheistic version of the twelve steps (see below).

Amma (*anma, pu tong an mo*): "General" form of Chinese Qigong massage based on acupuncture principles, including 361 "energy points" (*tsubos*). *An* means "press"; *mo* means "rub"; and *an mo* means "massage." The goals of amma include relaxation, improvement of blood circulation, and prevention of illness. Shiatsu (see below) stems partly from amma.

Amma therapy®: "Healing" system, developed by Korean-born Tina Sohn in the 1960s, that involves bodywork, diet, vitamin supplements, and herbs. It supposedly uses "powerful energetic points" discovered by Sohn; treats the "physical body," "bio-energy," and the emotions; and frees the mind and spirit. Sohn and her husband, Robert Sohn, Ph.D., founded and direct The Wholistic Health Center (WHC), an outpatient clinic in Syosset, New York. Robert Sohn, an acupuncturist and "master herbalist," founded and chairs The New Center for Wholistic Health Education and Research, which shares WHC's address. The New Center offers a three-year acupuncture program, an eighteen-month certificate program in massage therapy, a two-year certificate program in "wholistic nursing," and a twelve-month "graduate" program in advanced amma therapy. In its catalog, the school describes itself as "nationally accredited" by the Accrediting Council for Continuing Education and Training—which is not a recognized accrediting agency.

Angelic healing: Meditation with the aim of securing the therapeutic assistance of angels. Its premise is that angels invisibly guide, protect, and heal people through "radiant energy." It may involve the auric massage technique (see below), channeling (see below), guided visualization (see "Creative visualization" below), the laying on of hands (see "Contact healing" below), and/or prayer (see below).

Annette Martin training: System specializing in clairvoyant diagnosis (see below) and involving Edgar Cayce techniques (see Chapter 7).

Anthroposophical medicine (anthroposophically-extended medicine): Ill-defined pseudomedical system based on the occult philosophy of Rudolf Steiner (1861–1925). Anthroposophists hold that the human organism consists of a physical body, a vegetal "etheric" body, an animalistic "astral" or "soul" body, and an "ego" or "spirit." Anthroposophical "remedies" supposedly smooth the interaction of these components. (For a detailed description of anthroposophy, see my first book, *Mystical Diets*.)

Applied kinesiology (kinesiology): Elaborate vitalistic system of pseudo-diagnosis and treatment centering on "muscle-testing." Detroit chiropractor George J. Goodheart, Jr., introduced applied kinesiology as a diagnostic method in 1964. Goodheart theorized that muscle groups share "energy pathways" with internal organs and that, therefore, every organ dysfunction is discoverable in a related muscle. Testing muscles for relative strength and tone supposedly taps the body's "innate intelligence" and enables practitioners to detect specific dysfunctions. Applied kinesiology may involve chiropractic manipulation, craniosacral therapy (see below), diet, and "meridian therapy." In *Health and Healing: Understanding Conventional and Alternative Medicine* (1983), Andrew Weil, M.D., wrote: "Applied kinesiology looks more like a parlor trick, and its enthusiastic use by holistic practitioners shows how uncritical they can be in taking up methods whose main appeal is their unorthodox nature." (In scientific medicine, the word "kinesiology" refers to the study of muscles and human motion.)

Archetypal psychology: Form of "psychotherapy" akin to theotherapy (see below) and promoted by Jungian analyst Jean Shinoda Bolen. Archetypal psychology focuses on myths as keys to self-knowledge. Psychiatrist Carl Jung used the word "archetypes" to denote hypothetical ultimate mental patterns that constitute a "collective unconscious" (see "Jungian psychology" below).

Aroma behavior conditioning (ABC): Combination of aromatherapy (see below) and neuro-linguistic programming (see below).

Aromatherapy: Use of essential (i.e., volatile, aromatic, and flammable) oils from plants, flowers, or wood resins to affect mood or promote health. The oils are sniffed, ingested, or applied to the skin, usually with massage. Although aromatherapy is rooted in antiquity, proponents did not call it "aromatherapy" before the 1930s. Time-Life Books' *Powers of Healing* states that René Maurice Gattefossé, a French chemist, developed aromatherapy in the 1920s. *The Arkana Dictionary of New Perspectives* (1989) states that French homeopaths Dr. and Mme. Maury revived it in the 1960s. *Mysteries of Mind, Space & Time—The Unexplained* (1992) states that the basis for the selection of flower scents is the "doctrine of signatures." This holds that herbs and other living things have a unique quality or "vibration" revealed in their shape and/or color. *Mysteries* explains: "In aromatherapy, the violet is considered a 'shy' plant because of the way it hides its flower heads among its leaves. So the scent of violets is believed to bring feelings of calmness and modesty as good effects." The scent of chrysanthemums supposedly "inspires mysticism, otherworldliness, and psychic abilities." Some practitioners combine aromatherapy with chakra healing (see below), chiropractic manipulation, color therapy (see below), or diet. The May/June 1992 issue of *East West Natural Health* warned: "Some books suggest taking oils internally by placing drops of them on a cube of sugar, but the sugar may prevent a person from detecting how strong the oil is and result in an overdose. . . . Some persons who identify themselves as aromatherapists have only had a two-day seminar training." In *The Complete Book of Essential Oils and Aromatherapy* (1991), Valerie Ann Worwood—who called her work the household manual of the future—stated that there were about three hundred essential oils and that they constituted "an extremely effective medical system." She also cited "the holy anointing oil that God directed Moses to make."

Aromics™: Combination of aromatherapy (see above) and neuro-linguistic programming (see below). It involves sets of videotapes, audiotapes, and inhalers allegedly designed to help users lose weight, quit smoking, reduce stress, or become energetic or enthusiastic.

Astanga yoga (*ashtanga* yoga, raja yoga): Alleged prototype of hatha yoga (see below) involving lifestyle and *ujaya* breathing. The latter supposedly "helps purify the cells and organs in the body."

Astara's healing science: Form of spiritual healing (see Chapter 5) reportedly involving crystals, "etheric contacts," scientific prayer, visualization, and the "magnetic energies" of "the White Light." Astara is a school that occupies ten acres in Upland, California, and offers a correspondence course in mysticism, esotericism, and metaphysics. Its brochure states: "Astara is a new age church of mystic Christianity, following reverently after the teachings of Jesus. Astara also honors and pays homage to the saints, sages and seers of all religions." A November 1993 mailing states that the school's sole purpose is "THE GOOD OF THE WORLD" and claims that "Astarian initiates possess more riches than the whole known world is worth." The school also teaches the "science" of lama yoga (see below).

Aston-patterning®: Derivative of rolfing (see below and Chapter 10) developed by Judith Aston. It involves manually moving connective tissue in an asymmetrical spiral and "movement education." *Hands-On Healing* (1989) quotes Aston: "The body wants to move in an asymmetrical spiral."

Astrologic medicine (astral healing, astrological healing, astromedicine, medical astrology): System based on "cosmobiology," a pseudoscience claiming that specific mental and physical conditions correspond to the relative positions of celestial bodies. Astrologic medicine involves horoscopic astrology and the "zodiacal man" doctrine. Horoscopic astrology (horoscopy) posits a relationship between the positions of planets and stars and an individual's moment of birth that determines lifelong personality. The "zodiacal man" doctrine holds that the twelve signs of the zodiac—constellations named Aries, Taurus, etc.—rule different parts of the human anatomy. Proponents associate these astrological signs with organs, other bodily parts, and predispositions to disease in the associated parts. Certain "planetary configurations" supposedly can trigger disease in susceptible persons. Astrologic medicine includes "astrodiagnosis," pseudoprognosis, the timing and selection of treatments (especially homeopathic "remedies"), and "preventive medicine."

Attunement: Lifestyle and manual "vibrational healing art."

Aura analysis (aura reading, auric diagnosis): Direct (imaginary) or indirect examination of an "energy field" ("aura") surrounding the human body. Proponents claim that the aura is perceptible to clairvoyants or psychics. "Nonpsychics" supposedly can analyze it through Kirlian photography (see Chapter 4) or a Kilner screen. Dr. Walter J. Kilner (1847–1920) of St. Thomas's Hospital, in London, invented this screen—two plates of glass, an eighth of an inch apart, containing an alcoholic solution of a dye (usually carmine or a coal-tar dye). "Auric" colors allegedly reveal the personal traits of the subject, such as avarice, generosity, strong will, sensitivity, stubbornness, playfulness, ingenuity, impressionableness, shyness, immaturity, obsessiveness, melancholy, masculinity, femininity, and "spiritual arrogance." Proponents also associate "auric" colors with organs (e.g., glands), organ systems, and psychological states such as anger and boredom.

Aura balancing (auric healing, aura healing, aura cleansing, aura clearing): "Harmonizing" the "energy field" ("aura") around a person's head or body.

Aurasomatherapy: Both a variant of color therapy (see below) and a form of chakra healing (see below). Aurasomatherapy, the brainchild of British clairvoyant Vicky Wall, involves pseudodiagnosis and "color bottles." These contain emulsions of essential oils, herbal extracts, and scents. Practitioners allegedly revitalize and "rebalance" the "human aura" by using the emulsions.

Auric massage technique: Adjunct to angelic healing (see above) whose purported goals are to cleanse the human "aura," to revitalize the central nervous system, and to restore harmony to the body by restoring harmony to its "subtle bodies" (see Chapter 3).

Auricular reflexology: Mode of reflexology (see below) whose focus is the ear. Dr. P.F.M. Nogier of France "discovered" the method in 1967. (See "Auriculotherapy" below.)

Auriculotherapy (auricular therapy, auricular acupuncture, ear acupuncture): Variant of acupuncture developed by Dr. P.F.M. Nogier of France. It is based on the theory that a set of points on the auricle—the outer portion of the external ear—represents a fetus (with its head near the earlobe) and that these points correspond to body parts. Such points number over two hundred. Diagnosis involves examining the ear for tenderness or variations in electrical conductivity. Treatment consists in either acupuncturing or electrically stimulating the ear-point "corresponding" to the anatomical source of the malady. The French and Chinese sets of auricular "acupoints" are markedly dissimilar. In 1984, the *Journal of the American Medical Association* published the results of a controlled study of thirty-six patients given auriculotherapy for chronic pain. The researchers reported that stimulating locations recommended by auriculotherapy proponents was no more effective than barely touching remote points with or without electrical stimulation. The experiment demonstrated that any relief produced by auriculotherapy would be due to a placebo effect.

AVATAR: "Belief management" course developed in 1987. It is supposedly applicable to problems concerning education, finance, occupation, and health. AVATAR's fundamental doctrine is that people have a natural ability to create or "discreate" any reality at will. This alleged ability stems from a hypothetical part of consciousness AVATAR refers to as "SOURCE."

"Awakened Life" program: One of psychotherapist Dr. Wayne W. Dyer's audiocassette programs for self-development. It allegedly can teach consumers how to attune themselves to a "Higher Power." Nightingale-Conant Corporation, which markets Dyer's programs, equates this "power" with God, "Nature," and the "Life Force." The company describes the "Awakened Life" program as "powerful medicine" that has been helpful in the treatment of cancer, "other 'incurable' diseases," and addiction to smoking, alcohol, and drugs.

Ayurveda (ayurvedic medicine, ayurvedic healing, Vedic medicine, ayurvedism): The traditional Hindu system of medicine and its variants. It encompasses aromatherapy, diet, herbalism, massage, and Vedic astrology. (See Chapter 5.)

Baby B.E.S.T.: Adaptation of B.E.S.T.—bio energetic synchronization technique (see below)—to infants. In *Baby B.E.S.T.: Infant Adjusting/Care* (1991), originator M.T. Morter, Jr., a chiropractor, states that the main objective of this variant is "the removal of segmentation imbalances to restore symmetry to the child." This allegedly "allows for an updating of the neurological responses to and from the brain." In *B.E.S.T.* (1980), he claims that, usually, the left leg of acutely ill infants is shorter than the right, and that this "configuration" indicates "reversed polarity." Morter adds that during treatment, the child "may be under duress as the polarity returns to normal." (See Chapter 14.)

Bach flower therapy: Quasi-homeopathic system developed between 1928 and 1935 by Edward Bach, M.B., B.S., D.P.H. (1886–1936). Dr. Bach, a London bacteriologist, held that unhealthy mental states were the fundamental cause of disease. He intuitively "discovered" thirty-eight "remedies" for such states. These "remedies" are "dilutions" of various wildflowers. *The Complete Handbook of Natural Healing* (1991) quotes Bach: "Providential means have placed in nature the prevention and cure of disease by means of divinely enriched herbs and plants and trees. They have been given the power to heal all types of illness and suffering." In *Heal Thyself: An Explanation of the Real Cause and Cure of Disease*, first published in 1931, Bach postulated that the "conquest" of disease depends mainly on: (1) "the realization of the Divinity within our nature and our consequent power to overcome all that is wrong," (2) "the knowledge that the basic cause of disease is . . . disharmony between the personality and the Soul," (3) "willingness and ability to discover the fault . . . causing such a conflict," and (4) "the removal of any such fault by developing the opposing virtue." According to the *Dictionary of the Bach Flower Remedies* (1984), the mental states treatable with Bach's remedies include hidden "mental torture," vague fears of unknown origin, intolerance, timidity, self-doubt, fear of insanity, failure to learn from past mistakes, possessive love, lack of interest in the present, a feeling of uncleanness, a feeling of being overwhelmed by responsibilities, melancholy, self-centeredness, "Monday morning" feeling, impatience, guilt, panic, martyrdom, shock, extreme anguish, proudness, apathy, and resentment.

Baguazhang (pa kua chang, circle walking): Form of "internal kung fu" that amounts to walking in a circle. Dong Hai Chuan developed the "art" in the mid-nineteenth century. It involves at least a dozen stepping techniques, such as the "chicken step," the "elephant step," the "snake step," and the "mud walking step." Proponents claim that the practice enhances overall health and stamina, lengthens life, and improves "*Qi* cultivation."

Balance therapy: "Medical system" developed by Arcadi Beliavtsev, the "spiritual father" of face modelling (see below). Balance therapy involves "diagnostic" acupressure, homeopathy, and medicinal herbs.

Behavioral kinesiology (BK): Variation of applied kinesiology (see above) developed by psychiatrist John Diamond, M.D., and described in his book *Behavioral Kinesiology* (1979). *Applied Kinesiology* (1987), by Tom and Carole Valentine, cites Diamond's definition: "an integration of psychiatry, psychosomatic medicine, kinesiology, preventive medicine and the humanities."

Biblical counseling (nouthetic counseling): Use of devotional instructions in the Bible to treat psychological problems. Proponents equate psychological problems with spiritual problems and claim that all such troubles are solvable merely by cultivating obedience to Jesus Christ. The term "nouthetic" derives from the Greek *noutheteo,* meaning "to admonish or warn." Promoters of Calvinist fundamentalism introduced biblical counseling in the 1970s. Hybrids of the fundamentalist approach and folkloric "psychology" have largely superseded biblical counseling. (See "Psychology of evil" below.)

Bindegewebsmassage (bindegewebsmassage system): Form of bodywork developed by Elisabeth Dicke of Germany. It is based on the acupressure notion that treatment of certain areas on the skin affects internal organs correlated with them.

Bio-chromatic chakra alignment: Use of "visionary tools"—products allegedly based on extraterrestrial science—purportedly to unblock the "energy centers" of the body. These "tools" include the "Bio-Chromatic Integration Device" and the Starchamber™. The "integration device" supposedly converts "deep space energy" to "human frequencies." The Starchamber allegedly filters, focuses, and amplifies the "life force energy" in any object.

Biodynamic massage: Form of bodywork developed by Norwegian psychologist Gerda Boyeson, based on Reichian therapy (see below and Chapter 3) and involving deep breathing and relaxation techniques. Boyeson "discovered" that "blocked energy" builds up in the form of fluids, which supposedly become trapped between muscles and nerves. Biodynamic massage allegedly disperses these fluids and activates intestinal peristalsis, resulting in the release of emotions.

Bio energetic synchronization technique (B.E.S.T., Morter B.E.S.T., originally called bio energetics): Pseudonatural, chiropractic variant of self-healing (see below) and polarity balancing (see Chapter 11). M.T. Morter, Jr., M.A., D.C., developed the method in 1974 and describes it as an "approach to non-forceful chiropractic." In *B.E.S.T.* (1980), he claims that an "internal force"—"Innate Intelligence"—totally regulates health, that "Nature" is "smarter than we think," and that the body "does not know how to be sick." (See "Baby B.E.S.T." above, "Energy field work" below, and Chapter 13.)

Bioenergetics: Popular offshoot of Reichian therapy (see below and Chapter 3) developed by psychiatrist Alexander Lowen. According to bioenergetics, the human body is an "energy system," energy must flow freely for health maintenance, and all body cells record emotional or "energetic" reactions. Proponents hold that these cellular "memories" are adaptable to healing and consciousness-raising, and that the patient releases them by screaming, crying, and kicking. Lowen rejected Wilhelm Reich's orgone theory (see Chapter 3) but posited a "life energy," which he called "bioenergy." In *Bioenergetics* (1976), he defined "spirit" as "the life force within an organism manifested in the self-expression of the individual." He wrote: "I regard soul as the sense or feeling in a person of being part of a larger or universal order. Such a feeling must arise from the actual experience of being part of or connected in some vital or spiritual way to the universe. I use the word 'spiritual,' not in its abstract or mental connotation, but as spirit, pneuma or energy."

Bioenergy (bioenergy healing): Purportedly natural form of aura balancing (see above) wherein practitioners allegedly act on magnetic fields.

Biofeedback: Variable method involving electronic monitors (for example, an electroencephalograph), whereby individuals attempt to gain conscious control over autonomic (involuntary) bodily functions, such as the beating of the heart. Although biofeedback is not a supernaturalistic technique, it is often an adjunct to vitalistic methods.

Biomagnetics (biomagnetic medicine): Form of "vibrational bioenergetics medicine"; a "drugless" system of pseudodiagnosis and treatment related to cymatics (see below) and promoted by Sir Peter Guy Manners, M.D.

Bioplasmic healing: Variant of magnetic healing (see below) that supposedly involves "bioplasmic energy." (See Chapter 4.)

Biorhythm(s): Pseudoscientific method for predicting human conditions and susceptibilities based on alleged cycles calculated from the person's date of birth. The system was developed separately by Viennese psychology professor Dr. Hermann Swoboda (1873–1963) and Berlin physician Wilhelm Fliess (1859–1928). Swoboda and Fliess posited two cycles: a cycle of twenty-three days, supposedly predictive of an individual's level of strength, coordination, immunity, and self-confidence; and a cycle of twenty-eight days, supposedly predictive of emotional changes. In the 1920s, Austrian engineer Dr. Alfred Teltscher posited a third cycle, thirty-three days long and supposedly predictive of intellectual performance. According to biorhythm proponents, "vital energy" is high on "positive" days and relatively low on "negative" days.

Biosonics: Sound therapy involving music, tuning forks, crystals, massage, astrology, mantras, and color breathing (see below).

Body harmony: Form of bodywork that allegedly stirs up "natural healing energies," uses the body's "inner wisdom," and releases longtime traumas.

Body integration: Process that purportedly contributes to the "release" of "chronically stuck patterns" from one's physical, mental, and emotional "bodies." Self-styled multidimensional entity "Ziaela/Dr. Salomon" offers this technique and equestrian transformational expression (see below) at the Healthspring Center in Sedona, Arizona. In a flyer, Ziaela states: "I share the same soul as Dr. Salomon, and as a higher aspect of that spirit in that soul, have taken residence in this body to fulfill my divine purpose on this, the 3rd dimension. I . . . experience myself on the other dimensions as a being on an extraterrestrial/angelic craft."

Bodymind centering: Form of meditation developed by Gay Hendricks, Ph.D., and Kathlyn Hendricks. In *Radiance! Breathwork, Movement and Body-*

Centered Psychotherapy (1991), they describe it as "a precise, step-by-step technique for solving life problems through contact with the Inner Self." Bodymind centering supposedly "reconnects" the "Inner Self"—"the part of us that knows how we really feel"—and the "Outer Self." (See "Radiance breathwork" below.)

Bodywork: Any modality that involves touching, manipulation, and/or exercise of the body. Bodywork usually also involves the supposed alignment of the body's "energy field" or removal of blockages to the flow of "energy."

Bodywork plus: Combination of shiatsu, Swedish massage, imagery, energy balancing, and other methods. (See "Creative visualization" and "energy balancing," both below, and Chapter 11.)

Bodywork tantra: Meditative derivative of both Zen shiatsu and chakra healing (see below) developed by shiatsu schoolmaster Harold Dull. It encompasses: co-centering, watsu [wat(er shiat)su], and tantsu [tant(ric shiat)su]. Co-centering is a system of "pointwork"—the handling of areas of the body that supposedly house particular chakras or acupuncture channels. In watsu, both practitioner and partner are in a large pool of warm water at breast-level. The practitioner performs such actions as rocking and leg rotation on the more or less floating partner. Tantsu takes place on a dry surface. The practitioner holds the partner continuously and squeezes, pulls, or fingers various parts of his or her body. (See "Shiatsu" below and Chapter 3.)

Bone marrow *nei kung* (iron shirt *chi kung* III): Method of self-healing (see below); an outgrowth of iron shirt *chi kung* (see below). "*Nei kung*" literally means "practicing with your internal power." Bone marrow *nei kung* involves: (1) "breathing" *chi* through fingertips and toes, (2) contracting muscles to force *chi* into the bones, (3) massaging one's genitals to release *chi* for dissemination throughout the body, (4) hitting various parts of the body (e.g., with sticks), and (5) swinging weights—up to ten pounds—suspended from one's genitals.

BRETH: "Breath Releasing Energy for Transformation and Healing (or Happiness)." Kamala Hope-Campbell, an Australian, developed this method, which involves "conscious breathing," "high touch," and a "sitter." "High touch" refers to touching as a means of "soul-to-soul" contact and creating a "sacred space" for "deep inner journeys." A "sitter" is someone who supposedly creates a supportive and "sacred" environment. BRETH allegedly releases emotional and physical traumas and "limiting thought patterns."

Bubble of light technique (bubble of light meditation): "Magical healing" method whose premise is that the unconscious contains a "magic place" where anything is possible.

Cabala (cabbala, kabala, kabbala, kabbalah, kabbalism, Qabalah, Qabbalah): Eclectic and multiform mystical system of ancient Jewish origin analogous to yoga (see Chapter 5). The basic cabalistic modes are speculative (metaphysical) and practical (magical). Cabala involves meditation, prayers, rituals, demonology, and "angelology."

Cayce/Reilly massage: "Holistic" method based on the Edgar Cayce philosophy. (See Chapter 7.)

Cellular theta breath (cellular theta breath technique): Variant of self-healing (see below) based on "the power of the Breath." Supposedly, "the Breath," or "theta breath," is "transformation energy."

Chakra breathing: Variant of self-healing (see below) involving supposed activation and harmonizing of the "energy centers" of the "subtle body." Its purported goal is the restoration of "natural energy balances." According to this method, respiration connects the body and "soul." (See Chapter 3.)

Chakra energy massage: Use of foot reflexology to "open" the chakras (the alleged "subtle energy centers" of the body) and facilitate "spiritual evolution." (See "Reflexology" below.)

Chakra healing (chakra therapy, chakra balancing, chakra energy balancing, chakra work): Any method akin to aura balancing (see above) and relating to chakras. (See Chapter 3)

Chakra innertuning therapy: System involving meditation, mantras, "alignment," dream interpretation, diet, and yoga. (See Chapters 3 and 5.)

Chan Mi gong: Meditative form of Qigong (see Chapter 4) based on Zen (*Chan*) and Tantric (*Mi*) Buddhism.

Channeling (mediumship): Purported transmission of information or energy from a nonphysical source through human beings. These persons—called channels, channelers, or mediums—are sometimes in an apparent trance during the alleged communication. The "trance" mode of channeling is called trance channeling. The supposed sources include angels, discarnate former humans, extraterrestrials, and levels of consciousness.

Chen style: Alleged prototype of tai chi (see below) combining gentle and explosive movements.

Chi kung meditation(s): "Art" involving breathing methods, posture, and the purported "cleansing" of internal organs (see Chapter 4).

Chi nei tsang (**Taoist** *chi nei tsang*, **Taoist healing light technique, internal**

organ *chi* massage, organ *chi* transformation massage, and organ *chi* transformation and healing light massage): System of "deep healing" involving the massage of points in the navel area—a purported "storehouse" for universal, cosmic, earthly, and prenatal forces. *Chi nei tsang* allegedly promotes rejuvenation in patients without causing burnout in practitioners. (See "Healing *tao*" below.)

Chinese hand analysis: Form of medical palmistry (see below); an alleged means of obtaining information on health, sexuality, vocation, and spirituality.

Chinese system of food cures: Anthology of dietary prescriptions set forth by Henry C. Lu, Ph.D., in *Chinese System of Food Cures: Prevention and Remedies* (1986). The appropriateness of specific foods for particular symptoms, conditions, and diseases is based on three classes of food attributes: "flavor," "energy," and "movement." The system associates "flavors"— pungent, sweet, sour, bitter, and salty—with different internal organs. "Energies"—cold, hot, warm, cool, and neutral—allegedly determine the ultimate effect of ingesting specific foods. "Movement" refers to the alleged tendency of different foods to "move in different directions in the body": outward, inward, upward, or downward. Lu recommended eating fifteen to twenty-five oysters with meals to cure tuberculosis of the lymph nodes and goiter—or one may use oyster sauce as seasoning if fresh oyster is not on hand.

Chirognomy (cheirognomy): Pseudodiagnosis based on the overall shape of hands (that is, the type of hand), the shapes of parts of the hand (palms, fingers, and nails), the size of the mounts (cushions) of the palm, and skin texture. For example, small, flat nails supposedly indicate a predisposition to heart disease, particularly if their "moons" are barely visible, and nails with furrows allegedly indicate weakness of the lungs, especially if the nails are long, wide, and curved.

Chiropractic: System of "drugless healing" devised in 1895 by Canadian-born Daniel David Palmer (1845–1913), an Iowa grocer, fish seller, and "magnetic healer" (see below). Palmer postulated that the "vital force"—which he termed "Innate"—expressed itself through the nervous system. Today, some chiropractors cling to this belief, some reject it, and some consider spinal problems an underlying cause of disease. Rev. Samuel H. Weed, a friend of Palmer's and one of his early patients, coined the word "chiropractic." (See Chapter 13.)

***Chi* self-massage (*tao* rejuvenation-*chi* self-massage):** Sequence of massage movements that allegedly strengthens internal organs, sense organs, and teeth. (See "Healing *tao*" below.)

Christian Science: Religion founded by Mary Baker Eddy (1824–1910), which contends that mind is the only reality and that illness, pain, and death are illusory. It holds that reliance on medicine is sinful. Christian Science "practitioners" engage in absent healing (see above) and allegedly can bring about resurrections.

Clairvoyant diagnosis (psychic diagnosis): Pseudodiagnosis supposedly performed by clairvoyance—the alleged ability to perceive things directly (such as remote objects or future events) that are impossible to perceive by means of the human senses alone. (See "Psychic healing" below.)

Color breathing: Variant of color therapy (see below) involving visualization, meditation, and affirmations. Proponents advise those seeking to correct or relieve a condition to imagine breathing one or several colors associated with diseases, material success, personality, or "spiritual attunement." The method apparently stems from a booklet titled *Colour Breathing* by Mrs. Ivah Bergh Whitten, which was published in England in 1948.

Color meditation (color magick): Variant of color therapy (see below) developed by occultist Ray Buckland and described in his book *Practical Color Magick* (1984). The meditator sequentially visualizes cones of different colors pointing toward his or her color-coded chakras (see Chapter 3).

Color projection: Form of color therapy (see below) purportedly of ancient origin. It involves the passage of sunlight or artificial light through colored sheets made from gelatin and cellulose acetate or from silk. The alleged physiologic effects of color projection supposedly vary with the color of the filter. For example, light passing through a red filter allegedly increases hemoglobin formation, and light passing through a blue filter supposedly eliminates or reduces fever.

Color psychology: Variant of color therapy (see below).

Color synergy: Theistic combination of color therapy (see below), creative visualization (see below), and prayerful affirmations.

Color therapy (chromotherapy, color healing, chromopathy): Treatment involving light, food, clothing, and environment, based on the belief that colors have wide-ranging curative effects. "Color therapists" claim that cures result from correction of "color imbalances." Many hold that the seven colors of the spectrum correspond to the seven major chakras ("energy centers" of the body). Modern color therapy is based partly on the teachings of two mystics who were interested in "auric" colors: Rudolf Steiner and Charles W. Leadbeater. The means of diagnosis and treatment vary from practitioner to practitioner.

Concept-therapy® (**concept-therapy technique**): Pseudonatural chiropractic system based on the notion of "Innate to Innate communication." Chiropractor Thurman Fleet (1895–1983) introduced it in 1931. It comprises suggestive therapy (see below) and suggestive therapy zone procedure (see below). In a flyer, the Concept-Therapy Institute describes concept-therapy as a workable and logical "philosophy of life" based on the "immutable Laws" of the "entire Universe." (See Chapter 13 .)

Contact healing (the laying on of hands): "Healing" by touching a patient with the hands or palms. Contact healing, at least fifteen thousand years old, is based on the belief that a healthy person has "vital energy" to spare, which is transmittable into sick persons. It allegedly cures arthritis, asthma, bursitis, cancer, cataracts, cerebral palsy, epilepsy, heart disease, paralysis, tooth decay, tuberculosis, vertigo, and many other conditions. Usually, the "healer" places his hands, palms down, on the top of the patient's head or on the shoulders or waist. Some proponents use the term "laying on of hands" interchangeably with "touch therapy," which refers to such methods as OMEGA, reiki, and therapeutic touch.

Core energetics (core energetic therapy): Form of bodywork developed by John C. Pierrakos, M.D., involving chakras and the "human energy field." It is based on his personal experience, Reichian therapy, and lectures supposedly transmitted through Eva Pierrakos by a "spirit entity" known only as "the Guide." Ms. Pierrakos died in 1979. Practitioners direct core energetics toward the integration of body, mind, spirit, and soul. Drs. Pierrakos and Alexander Lowen cofounded the Institute for Bioenergetic Analysis, but Pierrakos left the institute in 1974 and later developed core energetic therapy. (See "Reichian therapy" below and Chapter 3.)

Cosmic energy *chi kung* (cosmic healing *chi kung*, cosmic *chi kung*): Variant of Qigong therapy and self-healing (see below for both) taught by the Healing Tao Center (see "Healing *tao*" below). A late 1993 catalog describes it as "a hands-on technique using acupuncture points in the hand, such as the palm, to activate and open acupuncture meridians throughout the body." The practice is purported to "cultivate, channel and mix the cosmic force with the saliva to nourish Chi."

Cosmic vibrational healing: Variant of astrologic medicine (see above). The major premises of cosmic vibrational healing are: (1) that humans absorb stellar energy, (2) that different stars have different effects, (3) that the brighter a star is, the greater its influence, and (4) that humans can attune themselves to particular stars either by meditating on them or by ingesting or applying "starlight elixirs." In *Starlight Elixirs and Cosmic Vibrational Healing* (1992), Michael Smulkis and Fred Rubenfeld describe their production of these "elixirs": "We use a Schmidt-Cassegrain telescope with silver-coated mirrors. The light of the star is captured by suspending a quartz bottle filled with extremely pure water directly in front of the eyepiece. The telescope has a clock drive that enables it to follow each particular star as it moves and keep it centered within the viewing field.... Inert gas devices are used to eliminate the possibility of negative thought form contamination. After two hours, this vibrationally altered water is placed within a light-proof container. Pure grain alcohol is added as a preservative for this stellar energy.... The original liquid mixtures are made into a stock concentration by adding seven drops of the mother essence to a mixture of pure water and 40% grain alcohol."

A Course in Miracles: Bestselling self-study program in three volumes comprising over a thousand pages, first published (as a photocopy of typescript) in 1975. Helen Cohen Schucman (1909–1981), a research psychologist at Columbia University, supposedly derived the work from "Jesus" between 1965 and 1972. Proponents consider the course "spiritual psychotherapy."

Craniosacral therapy (cranial technique, cranial osteopathy, craniopathy, craniosacral balancing, craniosacral work, cranial work): Method allegedly involving manual alignment of skull bones—which, in fact, are fused and not "adjustable." The purported goal is to remove impediments to the patient's "energy." The "therapist" holds the skull in his hand and supposedly attunes himself to the patient's "rhythm." Proponents claim that movements of the skull bones cause movements of the sacrum and vice versa. They also claim that about 95 percent of people suffer from misalignment of cranial bones, which allegedly causes toothaches, migraines, and neurological disturbances. (See Chapter 9.)

Creative visualization: "Healing" system developed by New Age spiritual teacher Shakti Gawain. Gawain defines creative visualization in her bestseller of the same name: "the technique of using your imagination to create what you want in your life." She further defines imagination as "the basic creative energy of the universe." Terms for identical or similar methods include: visualization, visualization therapy, guided visualization, imagery, guided imagery, guided fantasy, mental imagery, active imagination, imaging, creative imaging, dynamic imaging, positive imaging, positive thinking, positive visualization, directed daydream, directed waking dream, waking dream therapy, led meditation, inner guide meditation, initiated symbol projection, imaginal medicine, imagineering (see below), and pathworking. In *Healing Yourself: A Step-by-*

Step Program for Better Health Through Imagery (1987), Martin L. Rossman, M.D., advocated consulting "inner advisors" or a "small voice within" regarding such matters as attitude, emotions, environment, exercise, faith, illness, nutrition, and posture. Rossman, a former student of acupuncture, said that such "advisors" come in the form of angels, fairies, gremlins, leprechauns, animals, deceased relatives, long-lost friends, the ocean, Winston Churchill, Mahatma Gandhi, Eleanor Roosevelt, John F. Kennedy, Buddha, Jesus, Moses, and the "Star Wars" character Yoda. He distinguished between "inner advisors" and "impostor advisors" ("inner figures" who are "heavily judgmental," punitive, and hostile). After one uses imagery for a while, he stated, "whole communities" of advisors may turn up. Rossman counseled against giving up the practice even if it worsens one's condition. "If you can make yourself feel worse," he explained, "you can probably make yourself feel better." (See Chapter 11.)

Crystal therapy (crystal healing, crystal work, crystal therapeutics): Use of crystals (especially quartz crystals) and gemstones to treat such conditions as blindness, bursitis, cancer, depression, forgetfulness, tension headaches, hemorrhages, indigestion, insomnia, Parkinson's disease, rheumatism, and thrombosis. According to the Winter/Spring 1993 edition of *New York Naturally*, an "alternative" healthcare directory, "Crystals draw light and color to the body's aura, raising its vibrational frequency to allow lower frequency energies to emerge for healing." Crystal therapy encompasses many methods. Its forms include aura balancing, chakra healing, color therapy, self-healing, acupressure, and radiesthesia. For example, a practitioner may place stones on and/or near the patient, sometimes on chakras (alleged "spiritual energy centers") or along acupuncture meridians. Some "therapists" use a carved quartz crystal with a smooth point for acupressure or one with a rounded end for massage. Other crystal "tools" include bracelets, coronets, pendants, rings, rattles, pendulums, and wands. Another method involves the ingestion of pulverized stones. Yet another involves placing a stone in liquid, leaving it there overnight or for several days, and then removing it and drinking the liquid. The liquid supposedly contains the "vibrations" of the stone. For self-healing (see below), proponents advise patients to wear, massage themselves with, or simply hold a suitably "programmed" quartz crystal, preferably along with "projecting" self-love. Some practitioners "diagnose" by dangling a crystal over a patient's chakras. Counterclockwise rotation allegedly signifies an "energy blockage." In *Crystal Healing: The Next Step* (1991), Phyllis Galde states that to use crystals effectively one must "turn off the rational mind." She recommends following one's intuition in choosing a particular method.

Cupping: Ancient method akin to moxabustion (see below). The practitioner uses either a suction device or a cup made of glass, metal, or wood and burns herbs, *moxa*, or alcohol-soaked cotton wool inside the cup. After the burning is complete, the cup is applied upside-down to a relatively flat body surface—for example, over an acupuncture point or meridian. The practitioner leaves the cup in this position for five to ten minutes and may repeat the process on different parts of the body. Proponents recommend cupping for arthritis, asthma, back pain, boils, bronchitis, pleurisy, pneumonia, rheumatism, and other disorders.

Cymatics (cymatic medicine, cymatic therapy): Form of "vibrational bioenergetics medicine" developed by British osteopath Peter Guy Manners. It is based on the notion that "life is sound" and involves audible vibrations that supposedly bring life to inert matter. Holding that every part of the body vibrates at a unique audible frequency, Manners invented a device that allegedly transmits beneficial sound to diseased organs when it is placed directly on the body,

Dayan Qigong (wild goose breathing exercise): Series of sixty-four stylized movements that purportedly imitate the postures and movements of the wild goose (*dayan* in Chinese). Proponents claim that the practice helps to delay aging and prolong life. They recommend it for gastrointestinal problems, heart disease, chronic hepatitis, hypertension, hypotension, insomnia, lumbago, neurasthenia (a neurosis), obesity, pyelonephritis (inflammation of the kidney), rheumatoid arthritis, skin diseases, and other ailments.

de la Warr system: Form of radionics (see below) developed in the 1940s and 1950s by British civil engineer George de la Warr (born George Warr) and his wife Marjorie. Warr invented a radionic camera that resembled a washing machine and a pseudotherapeutic "colourscope" that emitted light of different wavelengths. The camera allegedly could produce photos of the "vital force fields" of objects and pictures of past events. The photographic qualities of the "force fields" of blood spots and tissue samples supposedly serve to characterize illness. Warr died in 1969.

Depossession (releasement): Outgrowth of past-life therapy (see below). Depossession is a form of exorcism (see below) wherein practitioners purportedly remove troublesome ghosts or "nonhuman" supernatural entities from human beings, usually by persuasion. The alleged nonhuman possessors include "elementals"—"nature spirits" such as gnomes (e.g., trolls), satyrs, fairies, elves, pixies, and nymphs.

Diamond approach (Diamond approach to inner realization): Mode of "psychotherapy" geared toward the "retrieval" of "essence" (see Chapter 4). In *Essence: The Diamond Approach to Inner Realization* (1986), A.H. Almaas states: "The work on retrieving essence is primarily wrestling with the personality until it relinquishes its hold and surrenders its position to the true master, the human essence." The author holds that loss of "essence" is the root of all personality conflicts.

Diamond method: Composite approach based on the views of psychiatrist John Diamond, who developed behavioral kinesiology (see above). Life energy analysis (see below) is one of its major components.

***Dian xue* (*dian xue an mo*):** Vigorous variant of *tui na* (see below). Unlike *tui na, dian xue* centers on "acupuncture cavities." *Dian* means "to point and exert pressure," *xue* means "cave" or "hole," and *an mo* means "massage."

Dianetics: One of the main techniques of Scientology, a religion founded by L. Ron Hubbard (1911–1986). The term is based on Greek words meaning "through soul." Proponents describe it as a pastoral-counseling method for locating and eliminating unwanted emotional and psychosomatic problems. The goal of dianetics is to erase traumatic memories ("engrams") through a procedure in which an "auditor" may use an "E-meter" (a device that measures changes in skin resistance to electricity), purportedly to help the subject recall traumatic events. Some "engrams" supposedly have their source in the "past lives" of subjects.

***Do-in* (*dao-in,* Taoist yoga):** System of "self-acupressure" akin to hatha yoga (see below), involving stretches and breathing exercises. Michio Kushi (see Chapter 6) introduced *do-in* in the United States in 1968. *Do-in* supposedly attunes and invigorates body, mind, and spirit and revives "stagnant energy."

Dreamwork (dreamworking): Systematic inquiry into or use of dreams for healing and self-development. In *The Elements of Dreamwork* (1991), Strephon Kaplan-Williams, a "mandala process" trainer, writes: "The Dream Source may show the dreamer which archetypal energies are most active in her, or a life situation, so they may be made conscious and dealt with." He defines "archetype" as "a cluster of energy and form inherent in existence." His "Dream Warrior Credo" begins with the affirmation: "I have no dreams, I am born in the night."

EAV (electroacupuncture according to Voll): Method of pseudodiagnosis and treatment originally based on the "Dermatron," a galvanometric device invented in the 1970s by Reinhold Voll, M.D., of West Germany. This and similar devices allegedly can provide information about the functioning of organs by measuring "electromagnetic energy flow" along acupuncture channels. Practitioners claim to treat "imbalances" thus discovered by electrically stimulating acupuncture points and/or prescribing homeopathic "remedies."

Eighteen lohan tiger/dragon Qigong: "Healing" method involving a purportedly "extremely rare" set of Qigong exercises. Proponents claim it promotes longevity and strengthens the immune system. (See "Qigong" below and Chapter 4.)

Electroacupuncture (electrical acupuncture): Electrical stimulation of "acupoints," with or without needles. Electrodiagnosis to localize "acupoints" may precede electroacupuncture. Proponents associate "acupoints" with a relatively low electrical resistance (see "Electrodiagnosis" below and Chapter 3).

Electrodiagnosis (electrodermal screening, bioelectric testing): Localizing of "imbalances" along acupuncture meridians with a device, such as a Dermatron (see "EAV" above), that measures changes in electrical resistance in a patient's skin.

Electro-homeopathy: Use of electric devices in conjunction with homeopathy.

Electromagnetic healing: Form of "acupuncture without needles" that purportedly involves "tachyon energy." In physics, the tachyon is a hypothetical particle whose existence is doubtful. However, proponents of electromagnetic healing describe "tachyon energy" as "life energy" and claim that "science" has "harnessed" it. According to the April 1992 issue of *Total Health*, a brilliant Japanese astrophysicist—unnamed—pioneered the therapeutic usage of "tachyon energy." A 1992 mailing from Tachyon Energy Research in Beverly Hills, California, stated: "After many years of dedicated research, the Japanese Tachyon Energy Institute has finally discovered a way to tap into and focus this energy from the air-space. Using a unique method of processing materials through an advanced electromagnetic field technology, they found that they could create materials that are highly organized at the molecular level. These 'highly organized' materials can then focus Tachyon energy." Tachyon Energy Research sells such "materials" in various forms, including mineral water, a moisturizer, clothing, and jewelry.

Electromedicine: Form of "energy medicine" that employs electromagnetic fields. It is based on the notion that "electrodynamic fields" control all living organisms. (See Chapter 3.)

EmBodyment: Form of aura balancing and chakra healing that combines sacred touch (a variant of craniosacral therapy), inner child therapy (see below), toning (see below), and other methods.

Empyrean® rebirthing: Variant of rebirthing (see below) based on the assumption that the breath has an "innate healing potential." Empyrean rebirthing allegedly increases this "potential."

Endo-nasal therapy: Variant of acupuncture involving the stimulation of points inside the nose.

Energy balancing: Use of firm, gentle contact between persons purportedly to facilitate the flow of "vital forces," rejuvenate the nervous system, and promote deep relaxation. Deep relaxation supposedly affords an opportunity for "healing energy" to dissolve tension and allow self-acceptance. (See Chapter 3.)

Energy field work: Any method or combination of methods involving aura analysis (see above) and aura balancing, with or without touch. Energy field work overlaps with bodywork and may also involve visualization and "therapeutic" conversation.

Enneagram system (enneagram): System of "spiritual psychology" purportedly of ancient Middle Eastern origin. It is based on the postulate of nine (*ennea* in Greek) personality types or primary roles: (1) the achiever, also called the reformer—rational, orderly, and self-righteous; (2) the helper—generous, possessive, and manipulative; (3) the succeeder, also called the motivator or status-seeker—ambitious, pragmatic, and hostile; (4) the individualist, also called the artist—sensitive, self-absorbed, and intuitive; (5) the observer, also called the thinker—analytic, original, and provocative; (6) the guardian, also called the loyalist—responsible, engaging, and defensive; (7) the dreamer, also called the generalist—manic and accomplished; (8) the confronter, also called the leader—dominating, self-confident, and combative; and (9) the preservationist, also called the peacemaker—easygoing and receptive. Each type has a "prime psychological addiction," respectively: anger, pride, deceit, envy, greed, fear, gluttony, lust for life and power, and laziness. These "addictions" include the Christian "seven deadly sins." Recognition of one's type supposedly is tantamount to "spiritual awakening." In *What's My Type? Use the Enneagram System of Nine Personality Types to Discover Your Best Self* (1992), Kathleen V. Hurley and Theodore E. Dobson state: "Through self-knowledge each person is then able to relate freely with self, others, the universe, and God." In the process of neutralizing the "prime addiction," according to the authors, achievers become pathfinders, helpers become partners, succeeders become motivators, individualists become builders, observers become explorers, guardians become stabilizers, dreamers become illuminators, confronters become philanthropists, and preservationists become universalists. However, in *Enneagram Transformations: Releases and Affirmations for Healing Your Personality Type* (1993), Don Richard Riso, a former Jesuit of thirteen years, states that contradictions among books on the enneagram by other authors have confused readers. In a footnote, he warns: "If an interpretation or application of the Enneagram does not clarify your own experience of people in the real world, it is not only relatively worthless, it is potentially dangerous."

Equestrian transformational expression (horseback to heaven): Variant of chakra healing (see above) involving "telepathic" horseback riding. (See "Body integration" above.)

Er Mei **Qigong (***Er Mei***):** Form of Qigong therapy (see below) developed in 1227 by a Taoist priest. "Er Mei" is the name of a mountain.

Esalen massage: Form of bodywork combining elements of Swedish massage (see Chapter 10), craniosacral balancing (see above), rolfing (see Chapter 10), Trager (see below), and other methods.

Esoteric healing (seven ray techniques): "Exact science" put forth by English-born theosophist Alice A. Bailey (1880–1949) in *Esoteric Healing*— the inspiration for the ray methods of healing (see below).

Etheric surgery: Variant of aura balancing (see above) and psychic surgery (see below). The "metaphysician" acts out an "operation" minus visible paraphernalia, allegedly treating the patient's "etheric body" or "etheric counterpart" (see Chapter 3). Physical contact is optional. Some forms of etheric surgery are also variants of absent healing (see above) or channeling (see above).

Eurythmy; see "Therapeutic eurythmy" below.

Eutony (eutony therapy, Gerda Alexander method): "Holistic" form of body-centered psychotherapy (see Chapter 12) created by Gerda Alexander. The prefix "eu" means good; "tony" means muscle tone. Eutony somewhat resembles the Alexander technique (see above and Chapter 10). The eutony model posits "blocked energy" and a collective unconscious (see "Jungian psychology" below). Eutonists categorize patients (called pupils) as hyper tonic, normotonic, and hypotonic.

Exorcism: Alleged expulsion of Satan, some other demon, multiple evil spirits, or an offensive ghost (discarnate human) from an individual or place by command or persuasion or through rituals, special prayers, spells, or symbolism.

Face modelling: "Aesthetic" form of massage therapy promoted as an "alternative to plastic surgery" by the Arcadi Centre in Amsterdam, the Netherlands.

The center's brochure states: "Non-conventional medicine frequently makes use of the fact that many internal organs are being projected on the skin of the face. The intensive treatment of your visage therefore implies that these organs receive a shower of healing impulses. Thus, a better physical condition appears to be a welcome bonus from Face Modelling."

Facial rejuvenation, a Burnham system®: Combination of massage—specifically, reflexology (see below) centered on the head—and "energy work." Facial rejuvenation allegedly increases "energy flow" to the shoulders, neck, and head; realigns facial muscles; and enhances inner harmony and healing.

Faith healing: Specifically, a form of religious "healing" wherein a "specialist" (usually a member of the clergy) makes petitions to God in the presence of the patient. Faith healing commonly includes the laying on of hands (see "Contact healing" above). According to some proponents, whether faith healing is effective depends on the degree of religious faith the patient possesses.

Ferreri technique: Variant of applied kinesiology (see above) developed by Carl A. Ferreri, a New York City chiropractor.

Firewalking: Centuries-old practice of walking barefoot across a bed of hot cinders (usually coals) or stones—or a pit of fire. It is usually a religious or quasireligious ritual. Many firewalkers ascribe their ability to deities, supernatural forces, or a personal "bioelectric field." The ability has been compared with self-healing (see below). In the United States, proponents have touted firewalking since the early 1980s as a way to overcome fears, doubts, and inhibitions and to develop personal power. Advertisements claimed that firewalking seminars could cure cigarette smoking, claustrophobia, chronic depression, gluttony, and impotence. In recent years, proponents have even praised firewalking as a model for solving global problems, comparing the "firewalk" to AIDS, cancer, ecological emergencies, and economic disarray. In *Dancing with the Fire* (1989), Michael Sky writes: "*Somehow a solution resides in the heart of each fire.* Ultimately, all of our paths lead...into the center of the heat." The Firewalking Institute of Research and Education (FIRE) in Twain Harte, California, offers a four-day "firewalking instructor's certification" program. FIRE describes firewalking as a "sacred ritual" and asserts that those who complete the program will continue to discover its "healing properties." In the Fall 1985 issue of *Skeptical Inquirer*, research psychologist William J. McCarthy asked: "What kind of people would pay $125 for the privilege of risking their soles?" First- and second-degree burns are not uncommon.

Flower essence therapy: Pseudotherapeutic use of liquid "extracts" from flowering plants. Richard Katz pioneered this sequel to Bach flower therapy (see above) in northern California in the 1970s. He wrote individual affirmations for more than a hundred "remedies." Preparation of "extracts" involves immersion of a flower in water and subsequent exposure of the liquid to sunlight or heat, whereby it supposedly becomes imbued with healing "life energy" and "spiritual elements" from the flower. According to *The Magical Staff: The Vitalist Tradition in Western Medicine* (1992), flower "essences" are made from hundreds of different plants. The means of selecting flower "remedies" include intuition and "muscle-testing" (see "Applied kinesiology" above).

Food combining (food mixing): Any dietary practice based on the notion that a meal's healthfulness depends partly on the compatibility of its components and/or the sequence of ingestion. (See Chapter 10.)

Foot analysis (Grinberg method): Pseudodiagnostic method "based on the principle that feet show us how we walk through life." Temperature, structure, and dermatological differences contribute to "diagnoses." Avi Grinberg founded the method in 1991 in Amsterdam, the Netherlands, and describes it in *Foot Analysis: The Foot Path to Self-Discovery* (1993). Grinberg claims that ingrown toenails indicate a proneness to headaches and that dry, tough skin on the outer side of the big toe indicates a problem with the upper cervical vertebrae.

Fusion meditations: Self-healing methods that purportedly convert "negative energy" into "quality energy" suitable for fusion with "positive energy." Fusion meditations posit chakras and a "soul body" or "energy body" (see Chapter 3 and "Healing *tao*" below).

Gem therapy: Wearing precious and semiprecious stones for healing. For example, in *Practical Color Magick* (1984), occultist Ray Buckland recommends bloodstones for hemorrhages and rubies for chills.

Gerson therapy (Gerson treatment, Gerson method, Gerson dietary regime): "A state of the art, contemporary, wholistic and natural treatment which assists the body's own healing mechanism," according to the Gerson Institute in Bonita, California. Gerson therapy involves sodium restriction, potassium supplementation, extreme fat restriction, periodic protein restriction, and coffee enemas. The institute promotes Gerson therapy as a preventative lifestyle and as a virtual panacea. In the Gerson therapy bible, *A Cancer Therapy: Results of Fifty Cases*, German-born Max B. Gerson, M.D. (1881–1959), described humans as microcosms of the universe governed by "Great Nature." (For a critique of Gerson therapy, see *Mystical Diets*.)

Graphochromopathy: Variant of color therapy (see above) involving the exposure of patients' photographs to sunlight or artificial light that has passed through an "appropriately" colored filter. The photograph should not include anyone besides the patient, and the diseased area of the patient's body should be distinct therein. The patient need not be present during "treatment."

Graphotherapy: Use of medical graphology (see below) to treat psychological problems.

Hakomi (hakomi method, hakomi therapy, hakomi body-centered psychotherapy): "Refinement" of Reichian therapy (see below) developed by Ron Kurtz in mid-1970s. The hakomi method supposedly uses the "mind/body connection" to elicit nonverbal "core beliefs." It is based in part on Buddhism, Taoism, and bioenergetics (see above). "Hakomi" is a Hopi word meaning: "How do you stand in relation to these many realms?"

Harmonics: "Transformative" and "curative" method of chanting developed and practiced by Tibetan monks. Proponents associate particular sounds with specific "energy centers" of the body.

Hatha yoga: "Physical" form of yoga that centers on postures (*asanas*) and *pranayama*—breathing exercises performed to control *prana*, the "life force." *Hatha* combines two words symbolizing *prana* ("upward-flowing energy") and *apana* ("downward-flowing energy"). Proponents claim that hatha yoga advances health, physical fitness, beauty, and poise, but they identify its ultimate goal as "self-realization"—supposedly attained through the awakening of a "great power." *The Sivananda Companion to Yoga* (1983) states: "Through persistently toning and relaxing the body and stilling the mind, you begin to glimpse a state of inner peace which is your true nature. It is this that constitutes the essence of yoga." (See Chapter 5.)

Hawaiian temple bodywork (*lomi ha'a mauli ola*): Variant of lomi-lomi (see below) that combines "prayerful" bodywork, music, the hula (a Polynesian dance), and breathing exercises for raising mana (the "life force"). (See "Kahuna healing" below.)

Healing light kung fu (healing hands kung fu): Technique combining cosmic energy *chi kung* (see above) and five finger kung fu. The latter is a set of exercises designed to process the "cosmic force" so that it "nourishes" *chi*. Healing light kung fu allegedly enables practitioners to channel "cosmic energy" through the hands for healing (see "Healing *tao*" below).

Healing love (healing love meditation, seminal and ovarian kung fu): Method of sexual intercourse that allegedly channels "sexual energy" into self-healing and converts it into "spiritual love." For men, it involves the "power draw"—sex without ejaculation (see "Healing *tao*" below).

Healing *tao* (healing *tao* system, international healing *tao* system, healing *tao* warm current meditation): "Subtle energy system" of self-development created by Mantak Chia, who was born in Thailand to Chinese parents in 1944. Chia directs the Healing Tao Center (also called the Taoist Esoteric Yoga Center and Foundation and the Immortal Tao Center and Foundation) in Huntington, New York. In 1989, a network of "Healing Tao Centers" covered twenty states and fifteen other countries. The healing *tao* encompasses bone marrow *nei kung, chi nei tsang, chi* self-massage, fusion meditations, healing light kung fu, healing love, inner smile, iron shirt *chi kung*, microcosmic orbit meditation, the six healing sounds, tai chi, and Taoist five element nutrition (all described herein). Chia and his wife, Maneewan Chia, describe the healing *tao* in *Bone Marrow Nei Kung: Taoist Ways to Improve Your Health by Rejuvenating Your Bone Marrow and Blood* (1989): "While learning to tap the natural energies of the Sun, Moon, Earth, and Stars, a level of awareness is attained in which a solid spiritual body is developed and nurtured. The ultimate goal of the Tao practice is the transcendence of physical boundaries through the development of the soul and the spirit within man." In June 1993, there were 189 active healing *tao* instructors in twenty-one states, Australia, Austria, Belgium, Bermuda, Canada, England, France, Germany, Greece, India, Italy, Japan, the Netherlands, Scotland, Spain, and Switzerland.

Hellerwork: Mode of bodywork invented in 1978 by aerospace engineer Joseph Heller, the first president of the Rolf Institute (see "Rolfing" below and Chapter 10). Hellerwork stems largely from rolfing and Aston-patterning (see above). Its components are rolfinglike massage, "movement education," and dialog ("talk therapy"). Regarding the third component, *Hands-On Healing* (1989) quotes Heller: "Over time I noticed that people started talking about certain subjects when I worked on certain parts of the body. That's when I realized that our bodies store emotions and attitudes. I've come to believe that these psychological aspects do shape our bodies." A course of Hellerwork consists of eleven ninety-minute sessions. According to *Hands-On Healing*, the theme of the ninth session is "how we express masculine energy," and the theme of the eleventh session is "how to allow full self-expression to radiate through the vehicle of your body." In an interview in this book, Heller stated how he helps people grow: "I work with what I call their channel for life energy."

Hemi-sync™: Audiotape system developed by The Monroe Institute in Faber, Virginia. The institute claims that particular hemi-sync tapes can control pain, increase strength, lower blood pressure, reduce appetite, weaken addictive behavior, hasten recovery from illness or surgery, enhance recovery of speech and motor skills after a stroke, and control the metabolism of food by either maximizing or minimizing "the caloric value retained."

Hippocrates diet (living foods lifestyle): Dietetic variant of self-healing (see below) that is the centerpiece of the Hippocrates health program (see below). The diet consists of seven categories of uncooked ("living") foods: (1) specific fruits; (2) specific vegetables; (3) fresh juices extracted from fruits, vegetables, and sprouts; (4) specific sprouts; (5) nuts and seeds; (6) fermented foods such as sauerkraut and miso; and (7) unfiltered honey. In *The Hippocrates Diet and Health Program* (1984), Ann Wigmore, the diet's originator, stated that "life energy" is the "active agent" of enzymes and claimed that the diet "stops unnecessary wastage of enzyme energy."

Hippocrates health program: Variant of nature cure (see below) developed by "wholistic health educator" Ann Wigmore, who founded the Hippocrates Health Institute in 1957. The program involves a vegetarian diet, food combining (see Chapter 9), enemas, deep breathing, brushing the skin, and exercises such as squatting. Formerly located in Boston, the institute occupies twenty acres in West Palm Beach, Florida. In *Hippocrates Health Program: A Proven Guide to Healthful Living* (1989), its codirector, Brian R. Clement, states that wheatgrass chlorophyll, food combining (see above), and the integration of body, mind, and spirit are "essential to optimum health." In *Belief: All There Is* (1991), he asserts: "People who have a belief that they are ill . . . will inevitably go from one physical problem or one disease to another until they ultimately pull off the biggest of all shams on themselves, which is death." (See "Hippocrates diet" above.)

Holistic dentistry: Form of general dentistry that may include acupuncture, biofeedback (see above), craniosacral therapy, and/or homeopathy (see below and Chapter 8).

Holistic gynecology: "Natural" approach to women's health that includes "vitamin and herbal therapies" and visualization (see "Creative visualization" above).

Holistic nursing: Form of nursing that exalts intuition. Its purported goal is "body/mind/spirit" integration. Often includes therapeutic touch (see below).

Holistic palpate energy therapy: Form of aura balancing (see above and Chapter 3).

Holistic reiki: Variant of reiki (see below) and form of chakra healing (see above) invented by interfaith ministers Marla and Bill Abraham.

Holotropic breathwork™ (holotropic therapy, holotropic breath therapy, holonomic breathwork, holonomic therapy, Grof breathwork): "Psychotherapeutic" technique developed in the 1970s by Czechoslovakian-born psychiatrist Stanislav Grof, M.D., and his wife, Christina Grof. Holotropic therapy involves breathing exercises, sound technology (including music), bodywork, and the drawing of mandalas—aids to meditation symbolizing the unity of the soul with the universe. One purported goal of holotropic therapy is to produce mystical states of awareness by releasing emotional conditions supposedly frozen in tissues. It is somewhat similar to rebirthing (see below). (See Chapter 12.)

Homeoacupuncture: Injection of "homeopathic solutions" into "acupoints."

Homeopathy (homeopathic medicine, homeotherapeutics): System of "energy medicine" developed by German physician Samuel Christian Friedrich Hahnemann (1755–1843). Hahnemann coined the word "dynamis" to refer to the "vital force." Homeopaths "treat" diseases with minute doses of substances—or with their alleged nonphysical, "quintessential" forms. According to homeopathy, the most effective remedy for a particular disease is that which can produce in a healthy person all the symptoms of the disease with administration of a significant amount. Hahnemann's final theory held that the "vital force" is the source of all biological phenomena, that it becomes deranged during illness, and that appropriate homeopathic "remedies" work by restoring the "vital force." In *Homeopathy: Medicine of the New Man* (1987), teacher and practitioner George Vithoulkas stated that one proof of the existence of the "vital force" is "the fact that when the disturbed organism of a patient is properly tuned through the administration of the right homeopathic remedy, the patient not only experiences the alleviation of symptoms, but also has the feeling that life once again is harmoniously flowing through him." (See Chapter 9.)

Homeovitics: Variant of homeopathy (see above) involving twenty-two formulations. HoBoN—"Homeovitic+Bio+Nutritionals"—in Naples, Florida, markets these and claims that applied kinesiology (see above) and electrodiagnosis (see above) can determine their clinical usefulness. HoBoN's catalog states: "Vitalized substances enhance detoxification by their transference of resonant energy to specific toxins in the living system. The toxin is then readily eliminated." For example, the company recommends two of its formulations for "detox" of "residual toxins" resulting from the ingestion of food additives. The "components" of these "detoxosodes" purportedly include "vitalized" food additives: citric acid, dyes, glycerin, mineral oil, monosodium glutamate (MSG), salt, sugar, sulfites, testosterone, and other substances.

Homuncular acupuncture: Any form of acupuncture centering on sets of "acupoints" said to represent a homunculus (a miniature human being). Proponents have localized such sets on the nose, face, hands, feet, and outer ear (see "Auriculotherapy" above).

Human energetic assessment and restorative technic (HEART): "Healing" method developed by George M. DeLalio, M.D. According to HEART, the brain produces "healing energy," "etheric pathways" contain this energy, and lifestyle and thoughts often disrupt the pathways. The technique involves "scanning" the "human electromagnetic field" for abnormalities and restoring the disrupted "pathways." (See Chapter 3.)

Hydrochromopathy: Variant of color therapy (see above) involving bottles filled with spring water or distilled water. These are either colored or encircled by colored filters. The user places a bottle with the "appropriate" color in direct sunlight, indirect sunlight, or artificial light and leaves it there for at least one to three hours. Then the patient drinks the supposedly "color-charged" water. For example, in *Practical Color Magick* (1984), occultist Ray Buckland recommends "red-charged" water as a pick-me-up and "blue-charged" water for fever.

Hydropathy (water cure): Internal and external use of water as a near-panacea (see Chapter 9). "Hydropathy" and "hydrotherapy" are not synonyms. In scientific medicine, hydrotherapy is a mode of physical therapy in which practitioners use water externally to treat specific ailments. Unscientific hydrotherapy includes both internal and external uses of water.

I Ching (*I Ging, Yi King, Book of Change, Book of Changes, Book of Metamorphoses*): Chinese book of ancient origin considered a tool of fortunetelling. It is part of the canon of Confucianism, the quasireligious philosophy that dominated China until the early twentieth century. *I Ching* combines two Mandarin words: *yi*, meaning "divination," and *jing*, meaning "classic" or "book." The *I Ching* features sixty-four hexagrams—drawings consisting of six lines each—which symbolize supposedly quintessential conditions such as innocence, tranquillity, humility, and happiness. All the hexagrams except one consist of both broken and unbroken lines, for example:

———————

——— ———

———————

——— ———

———————

———————

The consulter of the *I Ching* calls forth the "relevant" symbol in a haphazard manner. The above hexagram represents opposition and means: "When there is opposition, it is lucky if it is a small matter."

Identity process: Adjunct to neuro-linguistic programming (NLP; see below). In its 1993 catalog, NLP Comprehensive in Boulder, Colorado, states that NLP consists of ten distinctly different models—"ways to progress in emotional, mental and spiritual realms, so our human spirit can 'catch up' with or perhaps surpass the technological and intellectual progress of the past century." The catalog describes the identity process: "This process allows us to use our limitations as a doorway to an inner core not reached by other NLP processes. Some people describe the powerful feeling state they experience as an 'inner essence,' some as a 'spiritual core,' or as a 'connection with all'. . . . .Any 'symptom' becomes a gateway to pervasive change that goes far beyond the domain of the symptom itself."

Imagineering: Variant of both creative visualization (see above) and self-healing (see below) developed by Serge King. King holds a "Ph.D." degree in psychology from California Western University—an unaccredited correspondence school in Santa Ana now called California Coast University. Imagineering's premise is that both prevention of and recovery from illness depend almost entirely on the degree to which a person acts according to instincts. In *Imagineering for Health* (1981), King declares that "all problems are caused by a conflict of ideas." Imagineering encompasses four general techniques: idea therapy, visual therapy, verbal therapy, and "emotivational" therapy. Idea therapy includes the repetition of affirmations, such as "I am immune to colds." Visual therapy includes "color imagery"—the visualization of eight colors King associates with psychological effects. Verbal therapy includes "sounding"—"the repetitive expression of sounds that may or may not be in the form of recognizable words or phrases and which may or may not have any meaning." Emotivational therapy includes self-applied therapeutic touch.

Imaginetics: Form of magnet therapy (see below) involving products distributed by Imaginetics, in Bayside, New York. These include pendants, insoles, masks, and cushions. The company recommends "north pole energy" for all cases of inflammation involving redness, warmth, and swelling; and "south pole energy" for muscular tension and glandular underactivity. A 1993 mailing stated: "In man's long search of a universal cure-all, none fits the description nearly as well as magnetic energy fields. . . . The magnet . . . provides the means to precisely regulate the activities of every cell."

Ingham technique (Ingham method): Popular version of reflexology developed in the 1930s and 1940s by Eunice D. Ingham, an American physical therapist. She derived her method from Dr. William Fitzgerald's zone therapy (see below), concentrating on the feet. (See Chapter 10.)

Inner bonding: Variant of inner child therapy (see below) developed by psychologist and author Margaret Paul. Those who practice the technique allegedly become "spiritually connected."

Inner child therapy (inner child work): Form of psychotherapy popularized by Texas-born theologian John Bradshaw, a former aspirant to the Roman Catholic priesthood. In *Homecoming: Reclaiming and Championing Your Inner Child* (1992), Bradshaw states that all children of dysfunctional families lose their "I AMness"—that is, their assurance that their parents or guardians are healthy, able, and eager caregivers. He recommends that victims of this loss or "spiritual wound" reclaim their "inner child" by reliving their developmental stages and finishing "unfinished business." He terms such reclamation a Zenlike experience. Toward this end, he suggests having conversations with one's "inner infant," writing letters to it and reading them aloud, and writing letters to oneself—with the nondominant hand—as if the infant were writing them. Through such methods, the "wounded inner child" supposedly evolves into a "wonder child," which Bradshaw describes as one's *"Imago Dei*—the part of you that bears a likeness to your creator." He states: "You cannot be in touch with your wonder child and not have a sense of something greater than yourself."

Inner self healing process: System developed by American-born clinical psychologist and author Swami Ajaya, Ph.D. Ajaya is a teacher at the Himalayan International Institute of Yoga Science and Philosophy in Honesdale, Pennsylvania. He differentiates between the "authentic" ("true" or "inner") self and the "false self." A flyer describes the former as a "radiant essence," the "core energy," the "internal healer," and the source of abundance, joy, vitality, wisdom, and unconditional love. The "false self" is purportedly a false image resulting from the world's shabby treatment of everyone. The inner self healing process allegedly enables one to "rediscover," "come home to," and "begin to live from" one's "true self." It involves "experiential psychotherapy," "complete self attunement," and meditation. Through "attunement" sessions, one supposedly receives the "healing light" of one's "inner self." (See Chapter 5.)

Inner smile: Relaxation technique that allegedly increases the flow of *chi*. Practitioners "smile inwardly" at organs and glands. (See "Healing *tao*" above.)

Integral counseling psychology: Variant of transpersonal psychology (see below).

Integrative acupressure: Variant of acupressure whose chief distinction is a technique called "acupressure lymphatic release."

Integrative therapy: "Psychospiritual" method based on Jungian psychology and psychosynthesis (see below for both).

Interactive guided imagery^{SM}: Allegedly powerful variant of creative visualization based partly on Jungian psychology and psychosynthesis (see below for both). The Academy of Guided Imagery, in Mill Valley, California, offers a 150-hour certification program in the method. Its co-director is Martin L. Rossman, M.D. (see "Creative visualization" above). The academy's introductory workshop covers "using imagery for diagnosis," "monitoring progress through imagery," and "the spiritual dimension."

Iridology (iridiagnosis, irido-diagnosis): Pseudoscience according to which the functional state of body components is discoverable through examination of the iris (the colored portion of the eye surrounding the pupil). Proponents hold that the iris serves as a map of the body and gives warning signs of physical, mental, and spiritual problems. They ascribe the modern version of iridology to Dr. Ignatz von Peczely, a Hungarian. Supposedly, von Peczely discovered the "iris-body" connection in his childhood, when he broke the leg of an owl and a black stripe spontaneously appeared on the owl's iris.

Iron shirt *chi kung*: System of postures, movements, and breathing techniques. It allegedly promotes resistance to disease and enables practitioners to absorb and discharge energy through their tendons. (See "Healing *tao*" above.)

Iyengar yoga (Iyengar style yoga): System of postures, *pranayama* ("breath awareness"), and yoga philosophy founded by B.K.S. Iyengar.

Jin shin do® **(jin shin do**® **bodymind acupressure™):** System of acupressure based on the book *Way of the Compassionate Spirit*, acupuncture theory, Taoist philosophy, and Reichian theory (see "Reichian therapy" below and Chapter 3). Iona Marsaa Teeguarden, author of *Acupressure Way of Health* (1978) and *Joy of Feeling: Bodymind Acupressure* (1987), developed *jin shin do* in the 1970s. Practitioners determine which parts of the body are "tense." According to *jin shin do* theory, stressful experiences cause the building of tension at certain "acupoints." To "balance" the "energy" of the body, practitioners hold the "tense" part with one hand and supposedly stimulate a series of "acupoints" with the other. Proponents recommend *jin shin do* for allergies, bedwetting, constipation, nocturnal coughing, ear infections, lung congestion, nosebleeds, hyperkinesis in children, and other conditions (see Chapter 9).

Jin shin jyutsu (jin shin jitsu): "Non-massage" form of shiatsu (see below) instituted by Jiro Murai in Japan. It involves either prolonged manual application of "pulse-taking" pressure to "acupoints" along just eight meridians or simply movements of the practitioner's hands over such areas without contact. The practitioner's hands allegedly function as booster cables. *Jin shin jyutsu* uses only twenty-six to thirty acupuncture points. It holds that "energy" can become trapped in these points—called "safety energy locks"—because of tension, fatigue, or illness.

Josephing: Form of bodywork developed by Spencer Burke and his wife Dawn Brunet. The term "josephing" is based on the name of a Native-American tribal chief, about whom Burke had a series of dreams in 1982. *Hands-On Healing: Massage Remedies for Hundreds of Health Problems* (1989) quotes Burke: "I open my work to manifest Chief Joseph's consciousness of love. Our bodies do the work of our spirits. If the body is in pain, it can't do God's work." In 1989, Burke and Brunet were the only "josephers" and normally charged $100 an hour at their office in New York City's borough of Manhattan. (I requested information through Burke's answering device in July 1993 but did not receive any response.)

Jungian psychology: Any form of "psychotherapy" based on the quasireligious theories of Swiss psychiatrist, "paranormalist," and reincarnationist Carl Gustav Jung (1875–1961), the son of a pastor. Jung was a disciple of Sigmund Freud for several years until 1913. He used the German word *"Heilsweg"* to describe his own school of "analytical psychology." *"Heilsweg"* combines the ideas of "healing method" and "sacred way" and means "journey of the soul." Jung's theories include those of the "collective unconscious" and synchronicity (see below). The "collective unconscious" he posited is an alleged inborn, symbol-ridden psychological bedrock common to all or much of humanity but varying somewhat from culture to culture. The terms "collective unconscious" and "universal consciousness" refer to a supposed "group mind" of sorts that enables telepathy. Jung distinguished between German and Jewish psychology and supported the antisemitic and racist Nordic Faith movement. He held that Odin, the supreme Norse god, possessed the movement's leader. In *The Nazis and the Occult* (1989), Dusty Sklar wrote: "Criticism for his aid to the cause of what he believed would be a 'Germanic, Jew-free psychotherapy' has now died down, and in the present atmosphere of receptivity to occultism, his ideas, books, and disciples are in the vanguard, enjoying great prestige."

Kahuna healing: The shamanistic system of the kahunas—traditional Hawaiian medicine men (shamans). Huna is the native philosophy of the Hawaiian Islands. Its current emphasis is on healing and alleged extrasensory perception (ESP)—also called psi, "psychism," "sixth sense," and "voyance." The literal meaning of "Huna" is "that which is hidden, or not obvious." The literal meaning of "kahuna" is "keeper of the secret." Kahunas are priestly practitioners of magic. They are supposedly capable of foretelling the future, reviving the dead, and controlling mana, the "life force." Some proponents use the terms "kahuna healing," "Huna," and "Hawaiian Huna" interchangeably.

Ki breathing: Combination of *tanden* breathing, massage, and a series of exercises called *ki-ren* or *ki* training. "Tanden breathing" refers to a method whereby one supposedly taps the *tanden* (*hara*)—the alleged seat of *ki* in the human body.

Kirlian diagnosis (Kirlian technique): Pseudodiagnosis based on Kirlian photography (see Chapter 3) and aura analysis (see above).

Ki-shiatsu®/oriental bodywork (ki-shiatsu/oriental bodywork therapy, shiatsu oriental bodywork): "Time-tested healing art" encompassing a variety of manual methods and breathing techniques that allegedly "balance-nurture" the "whole person." Proponents claim that ki-shiatsu/oriental bodywork can improve circulation and vitality, release physical and mental restrictions, relieve pain, and strengthen the immune and digestive systems.

Kneipping (Kneipp cure, Kneipp therapies, *Kneipptherapie*): Hydropathy-centered system of "natural healing" promoted by Father Sebastian Kneipp (1821–1897) and by the Kneipp Institute in Germany. According to the newsletter of ANTHA (the Anthroposophical Therapy and Hygiene Association), in 1993 one town in Germany had five hundred establishments offering Kneipp therapies. (See "Hydropathy" above and Chapter 8.)

Kofutu system of spiritual healing and development: Variant of aura balancing (see above) that includes a form of "touch therapy" and a form of absent healing (see above). Its purported goals are to balance karma and to enhance the "spiritual creative faculty." (See Chapters 5 and 11.)

Kripalu bodywork: Form of bodywork based on kripalu yoga (see below).

Kripalu yoga: Variant of hatha yoga (see above) emphasizing meditation (see Chapter 5).

Kriya yoga: School of yoga fostered by Paramahansa Yogananda (1893–1952). (See Chapter 5.)

Kulkarni naturopathy: Ayurvedic mode of naturopathy (see Chapter 8) developed and named about sixty years ago by Indian-born V.M. Kulkarni. It involves a "natural food" diet, fasting, hypnotism, magnetic healing (see below), massage ("mechano-therapy"), sunbathing, *pranayama* ("psychic breathing exercise"), and yogic postures. (The term "mechanotherapy" refers both to manual treatment—especially manual treatment that involves a tool such as a vibrator—and to treatment with exercise machines.)

Kum nye (*kum nye* relaxation): "Natural healing" system, based partly on Tibetan medicine (see below), involving slow movements, posture, breathing exercises, and self-massage. It allegedly "penetrates" negative patterns and "constrictions to natural energy flow" and enables the tapping of the "energies" thus released.

Lama yoga: Technique that supposedly safely "awakens" kundalini (see Chapter 5), facilitates union with the "High Self," and promotes physical health.

Lane system of multilayer bioenergy analysis and nutrition (the Lane system of 3-dimensional bioenergy analysis and nutritional healing): Variant of applied kinesiology (see above) concocted by Robert J. Lane, a licensed massage therapist and self-styled bioenergy consultant. The Lane system features "3-dimensional chi analysis" of the alleged one hundred "bioenergy layers" of the human body, an expanded version of the LePore technique (see below), "advanced dowsing" (radiesthesia without instruments), aura balancing, "chi balancing," and dietary evaluation. Lane, who holds a B.A. degree in psychology, also offers Swedish massage in his Manhattan office. He illustrates "chi balancing" in his "manual for new clients": "Apparently the body senses 'vitamin chi' when it's within the energy field, signaling recognition of 'the right stuff' with strong muscle response. . . . Weak thyroid chi balancers include B-complex, iron, apples, olives, selenium, garlic, dark green colors." Lane sells the vitamin and mineral supplements, herbs, and homeopathic preparations used in his system. They cost from $60 to $120 for a forty-day supply. In his "manual," Lane states that his stock of such products "roughly equals a small health food store." (See "Radiesthesia" below.)

L'Chaim **yoga:** Judaic variant of kripalu yoga (see above). It involves chakra healing (see above), Jewish melodies, and *makko-ho* (see below).

Lemonade diet (master cleanser, lemon cleansing): One of the three major components of a theistic and vitalistic system of "natural healing" developed by Stanley Burroughs. According to the lemonade diet, the ailing person ingests six to twelve ten-ounce glassfuls of a special drink daily—and nothing else— for ten to forty or more days. The drink consists of lemon or lime juice, maple syrup, cayenne (red) pepper, and water. In *Healing for the Age of Enlightenment* (1976), Burroughs claimed that lemons have "unique anionic properties to produce or create the energy needed to keep the body in normal health." He recommended the diet for asthma, atherosclerosis, the flu, gastric ulcers, skin disorders—"for all acute and chronic conditions." (See "Vita flex" below.)

LePore technique: Form of applied kinesiology (see above) developed by naturopath Donald LePore.

LeShan psychic training: System that allegedly promotes a faculty for psychic healing (see below) through attainment of an altered state of consciousness.

Life energy analysis: Technique developed by psychiatrist John Diamond, the inventor of behavioral kinesiology (see above). Diamond associates acupuncture meridians with emotional states; "acupoints" with "particular aspects" of these states; and specific affirmations, bodily movements, tunes, and nutrients with these "aspects."

Life force balancing: Combination of psychic healing (see below), the laying on of hands, psychological "adjustments," and spiritual counseling developed by Barbara West, who practices in New York State. It involves a "healing science" called "intercellular regeneration."

Life impressions bodywork: "Healing process" developed by Donald Van Howten (also known as Ravi Dos) involving soft-tissue "restructuring," "subtle fluid balancing," craniosacral therapy, imagery, ayurvedic principles, and Hakomi "psychotherapy." According to "life impressions," human beings are spirits in physical form and human bodies ("idea bodies") partially consist of a "historic imprint"—experiences stored in body tissues. The purported goal of life impressions bodywork is to "update" imprinted tissues by releasing "bound beliefs" and "energy."

Light work: Form of aura balancing (see above) purportedly involving "spiritual guides."

Living foods lifestyle: Dietetic variant of self-healing (see below) developed by Ann Wigmore (see "Hippocrates diet and health program" above).

Lomi-lomi: Form of deep-tissue massage practiced by kahunas (see above) involving the laying on of hands. Practitioners also use their elbows and forearms.

Macrobiotics: Quasireligious movement and health-centered lifestyle founded by George Ohsawa (1893–1966). (See Chapter 6. *Mystical Diets* features an account of my attendance at a Kushi Institute seminar.)

Magical diet(s): System of "food magic" devised by freelance writer Scott Cunningham. In *The Magic in Food: Legends, Lore, and Spellwork* (1991), Cunningham holds that different foods "harbor" different "magical energies" and that "ritually preparing and eating specific foods is an effective method of enhancing and improving our lives." In a section titled "The Magical Uses of Junk Food," he recommends canned chili, iced tea, Coca-Cola, and Pepsi for "magical and physical energy." However, in the chapter titled "Health and Healing," Cunningham advises: "Avoid all fad diets." (See "Magical herbalism" below.)

Magical herbalism: Branch of herbalism propounded by freelance writer Scott Cunningham in *Magical Herbalism* (1983). Cunningham defines herbs as "magical substances, infused with the energy of the Earth." Magical herbalism includes forms of absent healing (see above) and amulet healing. For the removal of warts, pimples, and other blemishes, Cunningham recommends a procedure that involves digging a hole, dropping a bean for every blemish into it, and saying something like: "As this bean decays, so my wart will go away." He adds: "This, like all banishing rituals, should be performed during the waning Moon." (See "Magical diet(s)" above.)

Magnet therapy (magnetic therapy, magnetotherapy, magnetic energy therapy, magnetic healing, biomagnetics, biomagnetism, biomagnetic therapy, electro-biomagnetics): Pseudonatural, pseudoscientific, and supposedly time-tested variant of self-healing (see below). Proponents depict magnets as sources of "nature's healing energy" and recommend magnet therapy for all acute injuries, Alzheimer's disease, cancer, cataracts, cerebral palsy, colitis, constipation, diabetes, diverticulitis, gastric ulcers, glaucoma, hypertension, hypotension, hypoglycemia, menstrual irregularity, migraines,

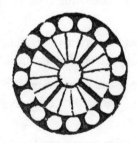

Mahikari "healing" symbol of planetary energy. The Winter 1993 *Journal of the American Reiki Master Association* states that practitioners wear this "divine emblem" in a pouch over the heart and that it "is never to be laid down upon the floor and is treated with the utmost veneration."

nervousness, schizophrenia, sinus congestion, and diseases of the adrenal gland, bladder, bone, kidney, liver, pancreas, prostate, spleen, and thyroid. (See "Imaginetics" above.)

Magnetic healing: Any pseudotherapeutic method that supposedly involves transfer of "vital energy" from "healer" to patient.

Mahikari: Trademarked spiritual movement and "healing" method founded in 1959 by Kotama Okada, a Tokyo businessman who claimed it was a product of "revelation." "Mahikari" means "true light" or "divine true light." Both as a movement and as a method, mahikari is akin to the radiance technique (see Chapter 11). Practitioners wear a "divine locket," which supposedly enables them to emanate and focus "light energy" through the palm of the hand. The method does not entail contact. According to mahikari, spirits wronged by ancestors cause more than 80 percent of human illness and unhappiness.

Makko-ho: Mode of stretching based on traditional Chinese medicine (see Chapter 4). It allegedly strengthens internal organs. ("Makko-ho" is a Japanese term.)

Manifesting (manifestation, conscious manifestation): Variable method for wish fulfillment that involves wholehearted visualization and positive thinking.

Manual organ stimulation therapy (MOST): Form of bodywork developed by George M. DeLalio, a chiropractor and registered nurse. According to MOST, "energetic imbalances" in particular organs are detectable through "reflex points" in the skin and the affected organs can be "reharmonized" manually.

MariEL: Method developed by "reiki master" and teacher Ethel Lombardi. MariEL supposedly is faster and more powerful than reiki. The term "MariEL" also refers to a "transformational healing energy" that allegedly works on the cellular level to help clients discover and "release" emotional and physical traumas.

Marma therapy (ayurvedic massage, ayurvedic lymphatic massage): Form of massage whose goal is to stimulate *marmas*—alleged vital "junction points" between mind and matter, which are invisible but palpable. Marma therapy may involve yogic movements and transcendental meditation (TM). (See Chapters 3 and 5.)

Medical graphology (grapho-diagnostics): Pseudodiagnostic method involving examination of a patient's handwriting. Proponents allege that handwriting reveals physical and mental illness. Some graphologists claim they can pinpoint diseases. In *Medical Graphology* (1991), Marguerite de Surany states that graphologists must consider nine basic factors: (1) letter shapes, (2) the shapes and locations of breaks in letters, (3) the shading of loops in letters or of the central part, (4) ambiguous letters, (5) superfluous letters, (6) omission of letters, (7) relative letter sizes, (8) unconnected letters in the middle of a word, and (9) variation in the shapes of particular letters within a text. Graphologists also consider the height, width, and slant of letters and the spacing between words and lines. De Surany interprets the letters of the English alphabet with reference to: (1) the twelve "organs" (e.g., "triple heater") of traditional Chinese medicine and (2) the meanings of Hebrew letters, Egyptian hieroglyphs, and Tarot cards. For example, according to the author, the letter "f" represents the small and large intestines—"both yang factory organs" whose complementary "yin treasury" organs are the heart and lungs, respectively. The intestines symbolize the "Minister of Finance": the small intestine sorts out waste and the large intestine either eliminates or retains it. Thus, an ink-filled lower loop of the lowercase letter "f" supposedly is strong evidence of constipation "due to a desire to hoard." (See "Tarot" below and Chapter 6.)

Medical palmistry: Application of palmistry—an offshoot of fortunetelling— to pseudodiagnosis. Palmistry comprises chirognomy (see above) and chiromancy (also spelled "cheiromancy"). Chirognomy is based on the overall shape of hands (that is, the type of hand), the shapes of parts of the hand (palms, fingers, and nails), the size of the mounts (cushions) of the palm, and skin texture. Chiromancy centers on the lines of the palm. Palmists also examine the hands for other marks and for colors. Proponents use the terms "palmistry," "hand analysis," "palm-reading," and "chiromancy" interchangeably. The purported goal of medical palmistry is to determine the condition of specific organs.

Medipatch™ healthcare system. (Medipatch™ system): Homeopathic spinoff developed by Robert Jordan and characterized by various Medipatch™ Homeopathic Remedy Kits, which are marketed for protection from low-level electromagnetic field radiations and such conditions as migraines and carpal tunnel syndrome (numbness or pain in the wrist and hand). Each kit includes "homeopathic" tablets for sublingual use, a medicine-carrying bracelet, and a "digitally-encoded homeopathic magnetic strip. In the December 1993 issue of *Body, Mind & Spirit*, Stephen Kravette, a naturopath and "professional astrologer" who works with Medipatch™ Laboratories Corporation, claims that the bracelet and "magnetic patch," when worn on the wrist or ankle, "interface with the 12 acupuncture meridian pulse points, strengthen the body's electromagnetic field (verified by Kirlian photography), and enhance the output of the chakral energy system."

Meditation: The act or process of giving continuous undivided attention to something. Various religions and quasireligious organizations promote meditation techniques as a means of achieving tranquillity and mystical awareness.

Mesmerism (magnetic healing): "Mind healing" method based on the concept of "animal magnetism" and named after Franciscus Antonius Mesmer (c. 1734–1815), a flamboyant Viennese physician who had originally planned to become a cleric. Mesmer theorized that an invisible, magnetic fluid permeated the universe, connecting human beings with one another and with the stars, and that disease was the result of inadequate supplies of this fluid. According to Mesmer, the task of the true doctor was to restore the equilibrium of the vital fluid among people. This he sought to accomplish with magnets, musical instruments, and tubs of water containing iron filings. Mesmerism was first debunked formally in 1784.

Metamorphic technique (metamorphosis; originally called prenatal therapy): Spiritual form of bodywork adapted from reflexology by Robert St. John, an English naturopath, in the 1960s. St. John formulated physical, psychological, and temporal ("time") maps of "reflex points" on the feet. He claimed that these maps involve personal experiences predating conception. Metamorphic practitioners allegedly communicate with the patient's "life force" or "innate intelligence" by manipulating points on the feet, hands, and head. Usually focusing on the feet, they supposedly act as catalysts in freeing the "life force" from genetic and karmic influences.

Microcosmic orbit meditation: Foundation of the healing *tao* (see above). It allegedly enables practitioners to connect with universal, cosmic, and earth forces; awakens and preserves *chi*; and circulates *chi* through the primary acupuncture channels. Purported benefits include the elimination of stress.

Middle pillar meditation (middle pillar technique): "Mental healing system" developed by chiropractor Francis Israel Regardie, who was born in London in 1907. It involves rhythmic breathing, chanting or humming, praying, and visualizing balls of light corresponding to five specific chakras. The meditator imagines these spheres emitting a beam of light—the "middle pillar." (See Chapters 3 and 11.)

Morter HealthSystem: "Complete system of chiropractic care" whose purported mission is "to improve the health of mankind worldwide." It includes bio energetic synchronization technique (see above), Baby B.E.S.T. (see above), a videocassette stress-management program called "The Twelve Steps to Stress Less," and nutritional supplementation "to restore the body to its natural alkaline state." (See Chapter 13.)

Moxabustion: Adjunct to acupuncture employing *moxas*—preparations of dried leaves from the common mugwort (*Artemisia vulgaris*) or the wormwood tree (*Artemisia chinensis*). Practitioners burn the *moxas* at "acupoints" to stimulate *chi*. They attach them to acupuncture needles, place them directly on the skin in the form of small cones, or place the cones on a layer of ginger.

Moxibustion: Application of heat to acupuncture points either in the manner of moxabustion (see above) or with an electrical heat source.

Mucusless diet healing system: Pseudoscientific method involving diet, fasting, eugenics, exercise, sunbaths, enemas, and bathing. Its developer was Prof. Arnold Ehret, a German-born Christian naturopath who died in 1922. Ehret set forth his system in a book of twenty-five lessons, *Mucusless Diet Healing System: A Scientific Method of Eating Your Way to Health*. He wrote therein: "The *Mucusless Diet* consists of all kinds of raw and cooked fruits, starchless vegetables, and cooked or raw, mostly green-leaf vegetables. The *Mucusless Diet Healing System* is a combination of individually advised long or short fasts, with progressively changing menus of *non-Mucus-Forming Foods*. This Diet Alone Can Heal Every Case of 'Disease'* [even] without fasting." Citing *Genesis*, Ehret proclaimed fruits and leafy, green vegetables the "natural food of man." Most other foods, according to him, are "mucus formers"—"wrong foods" that "contain, produce and encumber the human body with the matter of disease." Ehret claimed that rice-eating was the "foundational cause" of leprosy. He further claimed that "masturbation, night emissions, prostitution, etc., are all eliminated from the sex life of anyone living on a mucusless diet after their body has become clean and powerful."

Natural Hygiene: A no-frills form of naturopathy.

Nature cure (nature care): Variant of self-healing (see below) whose most important measures are fasting and rest. Nature cure was originally a hydropathy-centered "natural" lifestyle. (See Chapter 8.)

Naturopathy (naturopathic medicine, naturology): Variegated system—vitalistic, lifestyle-oriented, and supposedly "drugless"—whose basic theory is that disease results from the violation of "natural laws." (See Chapter 8.)

NETWORK: Chiropractic technique that allegedly uses "innate intelligence." (See Chapter 13.)

Neural organization technique (NOT): Variant of cranial osteopathy (see above) developed by Carl A. Ferreri, D.C. (see above).

Neuro-linguistic programming (NLP, neurolinguistics): Behavior-modification technique based on an alleged reciprocal relationship between physiology and vocal tone, posture, and eye movements. Richard Bandler and John Grinder initially formulated NLP in 1975, reputedly duplicating the "magical results" of several top communicators and therapists. (One of these was Milton H. Erickson, M.D., the originator of Ericksonian hypnotherapy.) The New York Training Institute for NLP lists NLP's "principles and presuppositions": (1) The meaning of your communication is the response you get, independent of your intention. (2) There is a positive intention beneath every behavior. (3) There is no failure, only feedback. (4) The map is not the territory. (5) People make the best choice available to them. (6) Everyone has the resources needed to accomplish what they really want. Advanced Neuro Dynamics, Inc., in Honolulu, Hawaii, offers a certification program in a style of NLP that "recognizes the importance of the human spirit and its connection with the mind and body." The company claims that its programs in NLP and time line therapy™—"an advanced NLP technique"— are "so powerful you may actually *feel your brain grow!*" The proprietors of NLP Comprehensive of Boulder, Colorado, stated in their 1988 mail-order catalog: "We're still amazed that we can often relieve a phobia, resolve grief or change a habit painlessly, in less than an hour—even though we have done it repeatedly and seen that the results last."

New age shiatsu: Style of shiatsu (see below) developed by Reuho Yamada.

Nichiren Buddhism (Nichiren Soshu, Nichiren Shoshu, Nichirenism): Japanese sect founded by Nichiren (1222–1282), a militant "prophet" who had allegedly been an early disciple of Buddha in a "past life." Adherents attempt to realize their wishes by chanting mystical words repeatedly, especially *"Nam myoho renge kyo"* and preferably in front of a rice-paper scroll (*gohonzon*) containing the names of "enlightened beings."

Numbers diet™: Reducing diet based on numerology contrived by Jean Simpson and described in *Jean Simpson's Numbers Diet* (1990). Simpson claims that by using numbers based on the dieter's last birthday, she can predict "the kinds of diet downfalls that are most likely to occur on each Diet Day."

Numerology: The study of the magical meanings of numbers and their alleged influence on human life. For example, numerologists associate the number eleven with the eleven loyal apostles of Jesus Christ; the number twelve with the entire group of apostles, the twelve signs of the zodiac, and the twelve months of the year; and the number thirteen—considered an inauspicious number—with covens (groups of thirteen witches). Numbers supposedly correspond to vibrations. Numerologists allegedly obtain information about the personality, capabilities, and future of an individual through calculations. These involve the letters of the individual's name and birthplace and the numbers of his or her birth date. "Unfortunately," according to *The Aquarian Guide to the New Age* (1990), "there are many different assignments of figures to letters. . . . Furthermore, the 'traditional' interpretations . . . can often vary widely." Numerological interpretation of people's names is also called "onomatomancy."

Nutripathy: Quasireligious system of pseudodiagnosis and treatment involving "spiritual" analysis of urine and saliva, food combining (see above), lifestyle, and a multitude of "dietary supplements." Gary A. Martin, an entrepreneurial, nontraditional Christian minister, developed nutripathy in the 1970s. Self-styled biophysicist Cary Reams devised the "formula" that is the basis of nutripathy. (For a detailed treatment of nutripathy, see *Mystical Diets*.)

Nutritional herbology: Part of the "educational" basis of Nature's Sunshine Products, Inc. (NSP), a multilevel marketing organization with headquarters in Spanish Fork, Utah (see *Mystical Diets*). Mark Pedersen, a "research chemist" for NSP, expounds on this system in *Nutritional Herbology* (1987) and *Nutritional Herbology, Volume II: Herbal Combinations* (1990). In the former book, he divides herbs into five categories "based on their active constituents": aromatic (volatile oils), astringent (tannins), bitter (phenols, saponins, and alkaloids), mucilaginous (polysaccharides), and nutritive (foodstuffs). In the second volume, he divides disease into "excess" and "deficient" conditions and explains the alleged utility of eighty herbal combinations partly in terms of the ancient Chinese theory of five elements (see "Taoist five element nutrition" below).

Ohashiatsu®: Combination of shiatsu, exercise, and meditation developed by Japanese-born Wataru Ohashi, who founded New York City's Ohashi Institute in 1975. The institute describes Ohashiatsu as a form of "touch communication" that integrates and rejuvenates body, mind, and spirit. Ohashiatsu practitioners supposedly discover the condition of their clients by feeling the *hara*—a portion of the abdomen below the navel considered a "spiritual center."

Oki-do: "Natural" lifestyle based on Taoism, yoga, Zen Buddhism, and traditional oriental medicine. It involves meditation, a "purification diet," and herbal "cures."

OMEGA: Method of "energy transfer," akin to reiki (see below), whereby practitioners simply place their hands on or near various areas of their client's body.

Organic process therapy (OPT): Form of psychotherapy endorsed for "rediscovering" one's body, feelings, mind, and spirit, and returning to one's "organic self." The therapist guides the client toward purported clarification of deep-seated physical and emotional problems. According to some therapists, such problems are traceable not only to childhood, infancy, and birth, but to "past lives."

Organismic psychotherapy: Spinoff of Reichian therapy (see below) developed by Malcolm Brown, Ph.D. In the 1960s, Brown collaborated with the founder of bioenergetics (see above). He divides human anatomy into four "ontological being centers" of the "embodied soul," which supposedly mediate distinct modes of interaction with the environment: (1) The agape-eros center—the upper frontal portion of the body—mediates feelings of openness toward others. (2) The *hara* center, which covers the abdomen, enables self-love and self-acceptance. (3) The logos center—the upper dorsal portion of the body—mediates "meaning-making." (4) The "phallic-spiritual warrior" center, in the lower back and four limbs, enables resoluteness (perseverance).

Orgone therapy (medical orgonomy, orgonomic medicine): System involving Reichian therapy (see below) and devices that allegedly siphon a deadly form of orgone. V. James DeMeo, Jr., Ph.D., founder of the Orgone Biophysical Research Laboratory, described orgone in an interview in the 1990 Flatland catalog of "small press" books and magazines: "It charges and fills all of the cosmos. It's what people in touch with nature have called God historically. You feel this life energy in your body when you go out to the beach on a beautiful day and you feel the energy in the air and in the water. If you're in the depths of the forest and you feel that the charge of life surrounds you, this is the life energy that you feel in your body." (See Chapter 3.)

Orionic healing system: Process that purportedly uses space-time and "God/Goddess as healer" and allegedly leads to profound release of emotional traumas and "negative thought patterns." Rebirther and hypnotherapist Janna Zarchin, M.A., co-developed the system.

Ortho-bionomy™: Bodywork method, developed by a British osteopath, involving dialogue, instruction in common movements, and, sometimes, purported manipulation of the "human energy field."

Osteopuncture: Variant of periosteal acupuncture (see "Acupuncture" above) using a different set of "acupoints" and, usually, a weak electric current. Ronald M. Lawrence, M.D., coined the word "osteopuncture."

Past-life regression: Use of hypnosis to explore the subconscious for information about alleged previous incarnations. Some proponents claim that the past-life regression can reveal information about the future (see "Past-life therapy" below).

Past-life therapy (past lives therapy, regression therapy, past-life regression therapy, transformational therapy): Mode of "psychotherapy" that emerged in the 1960s, based on a belief in reincarnation and usually involving hypnotism. Past-life "therapists" allegedly trace the causes of present physical and psychological problems to traumatic events the patient experienced in past lives. Proponents recommend past-life therapy especially for asthma, chronic back pain, chronic guilt, compulsions, phobias, and relationship difficulties.

Pathwork: "Spiritual" process including core energetics and based on material allegedly acquired through channeling—principally that provided by Eva Pierrakos between 1957 and 1979. (See "Channeling" and "Core energetics," both above.)

Pealeism: The Christian philosophy of Rev. Dr. Norman Vincent Peale, author of *The Power of Positive Thinking* and *The Amazing Results of Positive Thinking*. Between its publication in 1952 and Peale's death in December 1993, the former book sold nearly twenty million copies worldwide. The cornerstones of Pealeism are positive thinking, avoidance of negativism, fervent prayer to a personal God, and visualization of goals.

Pendular diagnosis (radiesthetic diagnosis): Pseudodiagnostic form of radiesthesia (see below) wherein the practitioner holds a pendulum over the patient. The technique is based on the assumption that diseased organs emit radiation different from that of unaffected organs. Supposedly, when the pendulum is above a diseased organ, the organ repels it; and the more diseased the organ, the larger the loop the pendulum makes.

Phoenix rising yoga therapy: Form of body-oriented psychotherapy (see Chapter 12) that involves hatha yoga (see above). Its premise is that unresolved emotional experiences are "stored" in the body—concealed from consciousness—and suppress the body's "natural freedom." The method supposedly establishes "inner balance" by "awakening" the "healing life force."

Phrenology (head-reading): The pseudoscientific study of human skulls to determine personality traits and mental capacity. Phrenologists consider the shape of the skull, the size and location of protrusions thereon, and hair growth.

Phreno-mesmerism (phreno-magnetism, phrenopathy): Application of the principles of mesmerism to phrenology. According to phreno-mesmerism, protrusions of the head relate to "cerebral organs" and their alleged characteristic emotions. There are supposedly several to more than a hundred and fifty of these "organs." (See "Mesmerism" and "Phrenology" above.)

Physiognomy: Fortunetelling and/or the purported determination of human character and disposition based on facial features or sometimes on the form and lineaments of the entire body. When the face is the object of physiognomy, the practice is also called face-reading. The "art" of reading the lines of the forehead is called "metoposcopy."

Pigeon remedy (pigeon therapy): Nostrum for jaundice rooted in rabbinical literature. The practitioner places a pigeon (dove or turtledove) on the navel of the patient. The pigeon and the patient are of the same gender. The bird purportedly absorbs all the jaundice from the patient and dies. Treatment sometimes involves more than one pigeon. Pigeon remedy and many similar folkloric practices are based on the notion that human illness (or sin) is removable to animals, plants, or nonliving things. Such practices have been called "transference treatment."

Plant alchemy (spagyrics): Form of "medical" herbalism based on astrological and alchemic ("parachemical") principles. One of the major goals of alchemy, a mystical "art," was to find the "elixir of life"—a panacea that could make humans immortal or semidivine. Plant alchemy holds that three "essentials"—termed Sulfur, Mercury, and Salt—constitute the basis of all matter. "Sulfur" is supposedly the masculine "world soul," "Mercury" the feminine "vital power" (*prana*), and "Salt" the material "vehicle." Spagyrists purportedly seek to extract these "essentials" from plants for use as remedies.

Polarity balancing (polarity therapy, polarity, polarity wellness®, polarity energy balancing, polarity energy balancing system, polarity system, polarity energy healing): Eclectic approach based primarily on ayurvedic principles. Polarity therapy encompasses counseling, craniosacral balancing (see above), "energetic nutrition," guided imagery, polarity yoga (polarity exercise), and reflexology (see below). Its originator, Austrian-born Randolph Stone (1890–1982), was a naturopath, chiropractor, and osteopath who retired to live in India in 1973. In *Your Healing Hands: The Polarity Experience* (1984), Richard Gordon states: "In polarity energy balancing, physical and nonphysical touch techniques are used to send energy through the entire system to open up the blocked points. This reestablishes the proper flow and alignment of life-force throughout the body." Polarity holds that the top and right side of the body have a positive charge, and that the feet and the left side of the body have a negative charge. Thus, practitioners place their right hand (+) on "negatively charged" parts of the client's body, and their left hand (-) on "positively charged" parts (see Chapter 10).

Polarity testing: Use of magnet therapy (see above) to determine treatment—for example, to select from such preparations as homeopathic "remedies" and nutritional supplements.

Postural integration: Form of bodywork promoted as a way of finding "a light, joyful balance with our mother earth" and of releasing and integrating "energy."

Prakrtika cikitsa (**naturopathy**): Form of naturopathy (see Chapter 8) based on the ayurvedic theory of five "elements": earth, air, fire, water, and ether (space).

Pranic healing (bioplasmic healing, radiatory healing): Set of methods based on the concepts of *prana*, "auras," and acupuncture meridians. (See Chapter 3.)

Pranic psychotherapy: "Simply pranic healing applied to prevent, alleviate and treat psychological ailments," according to *Pranic Psychotherapy* (1993)— "paranormalist" Choa Kok Sui's sequel to *Pranic Healing* (1990). Proponents recommend pranic psychotherapy for compulsive behavior, depression, drug addiction, hysteria, impotence, suicidal tendencies, and other problems (see Chapter 3).

Prayer (metaphysical healing): "Conveyance" of sentiments to a supernatural focus of worship or veneration (e.g., thanksgiving). Petitionary prayer involves a request. The two types of petitionary prayer are personal prayer and intercessory prayer. The petitioner is the intended beneficiary of personal prayer, whereas others are the targets of intercessory prayer. In Roman Catholicism, "intercessory prayer" may also refer to a prayer by which one asks a saint or similar deceased person to intercede with God.

Primal therapy: "Psychotherapeutic" method developed by child psychologist Arthur Janov, author of *The Primal Scream* (1970). Primal therapists dispense with analysis and attempt to resolve neuroses through a process of painful catharsis. Janov maintained that to be effective, psychotherapy must uncover repressed "primal pains"—unpleasant events undergone not only during childhood and infancy, but even in the fetal and embryonic stages. According to Janov, patients can dispel "primal pains" only by reexperiencing them and giving them physical expression (e.g., through screaming). The crux of primal therapy is rebirthing (see below).

Process psychology (process oriented psychology): Meditative form of psychology promoted by therapist Arnold Mindell, Ph.D. It involves bodywork, dreamwork (see above), spirituality, and the concept of the "dreambody."

Progression/regression therapy: Variant of past-life therapy (see above).

Psionic medicine (psionics): Offshoot of pendular diagnosis (see above) and radionic therapy (see below) developed by Dr. George Laurence. Psionic medicine involves the homeopathic concept of "miasms," treatment selection by means of a pendulum, and the correlation of diseases with colors. According to Laurence, health is "a balanced harmonious behavior of energy patterns." Homeopathy's founder, Samuel Hahnemann, coined the term "miasms" to refer to the three hereditary sources he posited for all chronic diseases resistant to homeopathic treatment. He labeled these alleged propensities "sycotic" (gonorrheal), syphilitic, and "psoric." "Psora," the original miasm, supposedly manifests itself as skin diseases such as scabies. It is analogous to the Christian idea of original sin—an alleged hereditary predisposition to evil. Some homeopaths reject the miasmic (or miasmatic) theory, while others adopt it uncritically and interpret it metaphorically. In *Radionic Healing: Is It for You?* (1988), chiropractor David V. Tansley defined "miasm" as "a specific focus or pattern of energy which will predispose you to certain diseases and symptoms." In psionic medicine, the practitioner places a blood sample from the patient on one side of a pendulum device, a "tissue sample" of "homeopathic potency" on the opposite side, and a proposed homeopathic "remedy" at the apex. The practitioner considers the "remedy" appropriate if the pendulum swings in a particular way. The word "psionics" also refers to radionics and "applied *psi*" ("applied parapsychology").

Psychic dentistry: "Miracle in the mouth"; supposed healing of teeth or gums, production of dental fillings in teeth, or generation of teeth by faith healing (prayer and the laying on of hands) or psychic healing (see below).

Psychic healing (*psi* healing, psychic therapy): Treatment by a psychic who supposedly draws "psychic energy" from himself, from spirits, or from God and then directs it through his hands to the patient, particularly to those areas "determined" by aura analysis to be unsound. It often involves the laying on of hands, prayer, channeling, or massage. "Psi" is the parapsychological term for the alleged abilities to become directly aware, without benefit of the senses, of events—past, present, or future—outside the body and to affect them without moving a muscle. Many proponents associate *psi* with prayer and meditation. Some allege that even animals possess it.

Psychic surgery: Alleged healing of diseased tissue, or its removal with either bare hands or common instruments, without leaving a skin wound. It is actually a sleight-of-hand procedure that involves palming and releasing a red liquid represented as "blood." Some psychic surgeons claim they operate only on the patient's "etheric body," or "perispirit." (See "Etheric surgery" above.)

Psychological astrology (astro-psychology): Combination of astrology and Jungian psychology (see above).

Psychology of evil: Christian "psychotherapeutic" approach propounded by psychiatrist M. Scott Peck, M.D. In *The Road Less Traveled: A New Psychology of Love, Traditional Values and Spiritual Growth* (1979), Peck equated laziness with original sin—an alleged hereditary predisposition to evil. Christianity ascribes original sin to an act of disobedience to God committed by the first human. Peck stated that the "lazy part of the self . . . may actually be" the devil. Moreover, he equated the unconscious with God. In *People of the Lie: The Hope for Healing Human Evil* (1985), which he called a "dangerous book," Peck claimed that he had "met" Satan. He wrote: "As well as being the Father of Lies, Satan may be said to be a spirit of mental illness." Peck used the term "psychology of evil" in the latter book to describe his goal. He explained: "We do not yet have a body of scientific knowledge about human evil deserving of being called a psychology." As a guest on NBC's October 12, 1993 "Today" show, Peck promoted his latest book, *Further Along the Road Less Traveled* (1993) and said he calls himself an evangelist because, on the whole, he brings good news. He also described himself as an "enormous admirer" of the twelve steps (see below). In *Further Along the Road Less Traveled*, he asserts: "Spiritual/religious ideas and concepts are necessary in the treatment of many people. . . . I realized that there was no way to treat . . . people [with phobias] effectively without trying to *convert* them to a . . . view of the world . . . at least as a place in which they . . . had some kind of protection in the form of God's grace."

Psychometric analysis (psychometric analysis of human character and mentality): Variant of radiesthesia (see below) developed principally by Dr. Oscar Brunler. It involves a pendulum device called a "biometer." M. Bovis, a Frenchman, invented and named the instrument sometime before World War I. He declared that all things emitted "waves" measurable with his device. Brunler, a physicist and engineer who died in 1952, "improved" Bovis's biometer and renamed it the "Brunler-Bovis Biometer." He "discovered" that a spot on the tip of the thumb afforded a means of estimating character and intelligence. In *Psychometric Analysis* (1959), Max Freedom Long recommended psychometric analysis for career planning and to determine individual morality. He stated that with psychometric analysis, "the subject cannot at any age . . . cover up his natural leaning to goodness or to badness—toward being constructive or destructive."

Psychometry (object reading): Purported means of acquiring information about people and events associated with an object merely by touching, handling, or being near to the object. "Psychic researcher" Dr. J. Rhodes Buchanan devised and named psychometry around the turn of the twentieth century. He held that all objects and events leave perpetual impressions in the "ether" or "astral light." Buchanan allegedly discovered that when psychometry students simply held drugs, the students often exhibited the symptoms that would have resulted had they ingested the drugs. Moreover, he allegedly found that some psychometrists could diagnose illness simply by holding the patient's hand. "Psychometry" literally means "measure of the soul." In scientific healthcare, the terms psychometry, psychometrics, and psychometric testing refer to the use of tests to measure such psychological variables as intelligence, aptitude, and personality traits.

Psycho-neuro integration (psychic healing): Method for "realigning" alleged "subtle energy centers" by integrating "subtle" and physical forms of energy.

Psycho-regression: "Unique" variant of past-life therapy (see above) developed by Dr. Francesca Rosetti. Rosetti's publisher, Samuel Weiser, Inc., claims in its catalog that her method helps people "find the cause of problems which may have their roots in lives lived hundreds or thousands of years ago." Psycho-regression allegedly releases "negativity" so that "positive energy and healing can flood in."

Psychospiritual holistic healing: Form of "psychotherapy" involving inner child therapy (see above), chakra healing (see above), meditation, and positive thinking.

Psychospiritual therapy: "Educational" pseudotherapy involving aura balancing (see above), guided imagery (see "Creative visualization" above), meditation, "philosophical discussion," and other methods. Its purported goal is the integration of body, mind, and spirit, which supposedly leads to "personal mastery."

Psychosynthesis (psychosynthesis therapy): "Psychotherapeutic" system originated in 1910 by Italian psychologist Roberto Assagioli and described in his book *Psychosynthesis* (1965). It is based on psychoanalysis and "Eastern meditative psychology." "Diagnosis" and treatment involve visualization and guided imagery (see "Creative visualization" above). Psychosynthesis emphasizes the "integrative powers" of the "superconscious" ("higher self"). One of its purported goals is to liberate and direct "psychic energies"—both "physical" and "spiritual."

Pyramid power (pyramid energy): In "alternative" healthcare, the use of "models" of the Great Pyramid of Cheops on the Giza Plateau to stimulate mental activity, speed the healing of wounds and burns, relieve headaches, promote restful sleep, and treat hyperkinesis in children. Both the Great Pyramid and "models" thereof—which may be open-frame or made of cardboard—supposedly accumulate and conduct "life energy" and "natural preservative energy" because of their geometry.

Qigong (*chi gong, chi gung, chi kung*, internal Qigong, Chinese Qigong): Chinese form of self-healing (see below) akin to yoga. It involves patterned breathing, posture, stylized body movements, visualization (imagery), and contemplation. *Gong* is a Mandarin word pertaining to skill. Its Cantonese equivalent is *kung*, as in "kung fu." "Qigong" literally means "to work the vital force" or "practicing with the breath." Interpretations of the word include "breathing exercise," "energy skill," and "energy mastering exercise." Qigong was originally termed *daoyin*. The Yoga Society of New York in Monroe, New York, calls Qigong "Chinese yoga." (See Chapters 3 and 4.)

Qi gong meridian therapy (QGMT): Variant of Qigong therapy (see below). The American Taoist Healing Center, in New York City, offers a certification program in QGMT and promotes it as a "highly effective natural healing system, used for a thousand years and still used today in hospitals in China." Its certification program includes "hands on training in Qi Gong Meridian Therapy and Medical Qi Gong for self healing and in the treatment of others." The center's flyer describes the supposed uniqueness of the program: "Special techniques will be taught to help the QGMT therapist increase and maintain personal Qi as well as to use it in treatment. The maintenance of good health and vitality is critical for any practitioner of TCM [traditional Chinese medicine], especially those who practice QGMT to treat patients. On the other hand, if the practitioner's energy is weak and unbalanced, it is not only harder to help patients, but one can actually make them worse. Secondly, as the patient's condition is often relatively unbalanced and weak, the practitioner must maintain a balanced condition in order not to be affected by the unbalanced Qi of the patient. Thirdly, as one uses some energy in treating patients, these techniques allow one to regain one's energy quickly." (See Chapters 3 and 4.)

Qigong therapy (medical Qigong, *Qi* healing, external *Qi* healing, Qigong healing, external Qigong healing, *buqi, buqi* therapy, *Qi an mo, Qi* massage, *wai Qi liao fa*, and *wai Qi zhi liao*): Treatment purportedly based on short-distance psychokinesis (PK), a form of *psi*. At most, Qigong therapy involves a light touch. *Buqi* means "spreading the *Qi*." "Wai Qi" means "external *Qi*" and refers to an alleged "shield" of *chi* at the surface of the body. *Wai Qi liao fa* means "curing with external *Qi*." In the Summer 1993 issue of *Qi: The*

Journal of Traditional Eastern Health & Fitness, Kenneth S. Cohen, M.A., compares Qigong therapy to noncontact therapeutic touch (see below). He states that the former method "may be dangerous to both healer and healee if the healer does not prepare himself properly." He explains: "If the healer is in a weak or vacuous state, then he may absorb either the client's diseased Qi or the client's own, much needed, healing Qi." Cohen further notes "the danger of a healer projecting his own diseased Qi into the patient." (See "Psychic healing" above, and Chapters 3 and 4.)

Radiance breathwork: Method comparable to holotropic breathwork (see above) without sound technology and mandalas. Psychologist Gay Hendricks, Ph.D., developed the procedure in the 1970s. He and his wife, Kathlyn Hendricks, a dance therapist, describe radiance breathwork and their other methods—including radiance movement therapy, radiance prenatal process, and bodymind centering—in *Radiance! Breathwork, Movement and Body-Centered Psychotherapy* (1991). Kathlyn Hendricks holds a "Ph.D." degree from the Institute of Transpersonal Psychology in Palo Alto, California, which was unaccredited when she obtained the degree. The authors state: "Therapy is about spotting all the ways you block positive energy and learning to let more through. Ultimately, if we let enough through, we become aware of our personal contact with universal energy, the divine."

Radiance movement therapy: Companion to radiance breathwork (see above) that allegedly "accesses the body's innate intelligence and allows long-held patterns of movement to unfold into new patterns."

Radiance prenatal process: Variant of radiance movement therapy (see above). Two practitioners—one male, the other female—support the client in water heated to womb temperature. They purportedly induce the client to return to the prenatal period, supposedly remove "troublesome" prenatal feelings, and perform bodywork, particularly on the head, neck, and shoulders.

Radiance technique®️ (real reiki®️): School of reiki (see below) promoted by Barbara Weber Ray, Ph.D., a clairvoyant astrologer who began using the term in 1986. The radiance technique is purportedly the unpolluted "science" of reiki's originator in its entirety (see Chapter 11).

Radiesthesia (medical radiesthesia, medical dowsing): Method of pseudo-diagnosis and treatment selection. "Radiesthesia"—literally, "perception of radiation"—is the anglicized form of a French word for dowsing coined by the Abbé Alex Bouly in 1927. Dowsing (also called biolocation) is a clairvoyant "art" centered on finding water, minerals, animals, missing persons, lost objects, or hidden treasure, usually with an instrument such as a pendulum or divining rod (a forked rod or tree branch, or a bent wire). The term "radiesthesia" refers both to dowsing in general and to medical dowsing—the use of dowsing to diagnose and treat disease. Bouly and two other French priests—the Abbé Alexis Mermet and Father Jean Jurion—pioneered medical dowsing. Mermet put forth his fundamental hypothesis in *Principles and Practice of Radiesthesia: A Textbook for Practitioners and Students*: (1) everything emits radiation, (2) "some kind of current" flows through the hands of human beings, and (3) holding appropriate objects renders them tools of revelation. The forms of radiesthesia he proposed include pendular diagnosis (see above), telediagnosis (see below), and teleradiesthesia (also called distant prospection). The assumption of teleradiesthesia is that radiesthetists can obtain up-to-the-minute information about a locality, geographic feature, or building merely by placing a pendulum above a corresponding map, photo, or plan. There are two basic "diagnostic" modes of medical radiesthesia. In one, practitioners supposedly detect and diagnose illness simply by passing their hands over the patient. In the other, they hold an instrument over the patient or over a sample of tissue or body fluid, a photograph of the patient, or one of the patient's belongings (such as an article of clothing). Practitioners of the latter mode base "diagnosis" on the movements of the instrument. *The Dictionary of Mind and Spirit* (1992) states: "Swinging to and fro is usually considered to have a neutral meaning; rotation clockwise and anti-clockwise are either positive and negative or vice versa. It is important to realize that there is no universal rule for this."

Radionic photography: Variant of Kirlian photography (see Chapter 3) developed by Hollywood chiropractor Ruth Drown, who was convicted of medical fraud in 1951 and subsequently died in prison. Drown called her version of radionics (see below) "Drown radio therapy." It included a form of absent healing (see above) termed "broadcasting." Drown maintained that there was "a resonance between the whole human body and each of its parts."

Radionics (psionics): Pseudotherapeutic offshoot of radiesthesia (see above) developed by Albert Abrams, M.D. (1863–1924), a San Francisco-born neurologist. Radionics encompasses radionic diagnosis (also called radionic analysis) and radionic therapy (also called radionic healing and radionic treatment). Abrams associated different diseases with different radio waves supposedly emitted by various parts of the body and even by tissue samples. After championing spondylotherapy (a system akin to chiropractic) between 1909 and 1912, he invented a pseudodiagnostic electrical system. Its components included: a "dynamizer"—a receptacle for blood or tissue samples, three rheostats—devices that regulate electric current, and an electrode, which Abrams affixed to the patient's forehead. Abrams claimed that one could even ascertain a patient's religion with his system, and further, that the patient's autograph could substitute for blood in the "dynamizer." For "therapy," he recommended his "oscilloclast"—a device allegedly designed to emit curative vibrations. In *The Medical Messiahs: A Social History of Health Quackery in Twentieth-Century America* (1992), Prof. James Harvey Young writes that while his "diagnostic" system was for sale, Abrams would only lease his hermetic "healing" apparatus, and then, only if the lessee had agreed never to open it. Inside was a purposeless configuration of electrical instruments and circuit elements. The American Medical Association called Abrams the "dean of gadget quacks." In *Radionic Healing: Is It for You?* (1988), chiropractor David V. Tansley stated that radionic practitioners analyze the states of "various aspects" of the patient's physical and "paraphysical" bodies. He further wrote that deepening knowledge of the chakras and the "subtle anatomy" extends the practitioner's capacity to heal (see Chapter 3).

Radix (neo-Reichian therapy): Offshoot of Reichian therapy (see below and Chapter 3). "Radix" means "root."

Rainbow diet: Vegetarian diet excluding "junk, fast, frozen, and irradiated foods" and based on "acceptance that all comes from God and is nourished by the God Force"—i.e., "OM, universal prana, universal consciousness, cosmic force, and virtual energy state." Gabriel Cousens, M.D., set forth the rainbow diet in *Spiritual Nutrition and the Rainbow Diet* (1986). "Animals may be our friends," Cousens wrote, "but they are not if we eat them." He claimed that "each food according to its outer color . . . can be related to the specific color and energy of a particular chakra" and that "each colored food energizes, cleanses, builds, heals, and rebalances the glands, organs, and nerve centers associated with its color-related chakra."

Ray methods of healing: System based on the "hidden meanings" of seven "formulas" that correspond to the "soul types" ("rays") of Theosophy, an eclectic religion. The rays, or "seven emanations from God," are a manner of categorizing people according to the purported qualities of their souls. The rays are: (1) willpower, (2) love and wisdom, (3) "active" intelligence, (4) art, beauty, and harmony, (5) scientific understanding, (6) devotion and idealism, and (7) ceremonial order or magic. Each associated "formula" supposedly indicates a method of "exoteric healing" (e.g., homeopathy), a method of service (e.g., white magic), and a method of esoteric healing (e.g., pranic healing).

Rebirthing (conscious breathing, conscious connected breathing, circular breathing, free breathing, vivation): A form of bodywork that employs hyperventilation. Leonard Orr developed rebirthing in the 1970s. Its purported goal is to resolve repressed attitudes and emotions that supposedly originated with prenatal and perinatal experiences. Practitioners—called "rebirthers"—encourage patients to reenact the birth process.

Reflexology: Ancient variant of acupressure. Reflexology is purportedly useful in assessing and improving the function of specific body parts. Proponents hold that all bodily organs have corresponding external "reflex points"—on the scalp, ears, face, nose, tongue, neck, back, arms, wrists, hands, abdomen, legs, and feet—and that manipulation of these points can enhance the flow of "energy." Reflexology allegedly can relieve asthma, constipation, migraines, sinus congestion, and diseases of the kidney, liver, and pancreas. The American Massage Therapy Association equates reflexology and zone therapy. (See "Zone therapy" below, "Ingham technique" above, and Chapter 10.)

Reflexotherapy: Form of homuncular acupuncture (see above) focusing on the feet.

Reichian therapy (Reichian massage, Reichian bodywork therapy, psychiatric orgone therapy; called vegetal therapy in Europe): Technique developed by Wilhelm Reich (see Chapter 3) involving bodywork and psychoanalysis. According to Reichian theory, blockages to the flow of orgone (a variant of the "vital force") cause neuroses and most physical disorders. Muscular contractions—"body armor"—in various parts of the body supposedly manifest such "blockages." The Reichian "therapist" intuitively decides where the greatest "body armor" is and seeks to "dissolve" or "dismantle" it. Efforts include massage and having the patient breathe deeply, gag, cry, scream, kick, make faces, and roll his or her eyes.

Reiki (Usui system of natural healing, Usui *shiko ryoho*, Usui *shiki ryoho*, reiki healing, reiki therapy; formerly called leiki): System founded in late nineteenth-century Japan by Mikao Usui (1802–1883), a Christian minister and Zen Buddhist monk who held a doctorate in theology from the University of Chicago. The term "reiki" refers both to "spirit energy" and to a method that is largely a variant of aura balancing and the laying on of hands. In *The Reiki Touch: A Reiki Handbook* (1990), "reiki mast ' Judy-Carol Stewart describes the "energy" as "pure God-force" that "flows from the universe into the crown chakra, the throat chakra, and the heart chakra, then out the arms and hands." This "love healing force," she continues, "has divine intelligence and will seek its own path in discovering and fulfilling the body's requirement." She distinguishes between "Reiki I energy" and "Reiki II energy" and states that practitioners can use the latter for absent healing (see above). The method involves touching parts of the body and "brushing" its alleged "aura" with the hands. The apparent aim is to transfer "universal life force energy" and thus effect healing and harmony. There are different schools of reiki, including that of the radiance technique (see above). The practitioner or "reiki channel" supposedly visualizes Sanskrit symbols. Students undergo one to four stages— rites wherein they purportedly receive "attunements" from "reiki masters." Proponents recommend reiki as a complement to acupressure, acupuncture, the Alexander technique, chiropractic, homeopathy, polarity balancing, and other unscientific methods. (See Chapters 10 and 11.)

Reiki plus® (**reiki plus system of natural healing**): Offshoot of reiki (see above) devised by "reiki master" Reverend David G. Jarrel and described in his manual, *Reiki Plus Natural Healing: A Spiritual Guide to Reiki Plus* (1991). Jarrel founded Pyramids of Light, Inc., a nondenominational "Christ-Conscious" church in Tennessee "dedicated to the laws of Natural Healing and the Teachings of Jesus the Christ and the truths taught in the Holy Bible." He also founded the Reiki Plus Institute as the "educational arm" of the church for "legal certification of Professional Practitioners." The "healing modalities" of reiki plus include: PSEB^{sm}—a form of aura balancing (see above); psycho-therapeutic reiki^{sm}—a method for releasing memories from the body, mind, and soul; and spinal attunement^{sm} technique (SAT^{sm}).

Remote diagnosis: Alleged paranormal discovery and rendering of the type and/or cause of a given patient's disease in the absence of the patient. Modes of remote diagnosis include channeling, clairvoyant diagnosis, telediagnosis, the de la Warr system, and psionic medicine (all described herein). (See Chapter 8.)

Rhythmajik: Quasicabalistic approach involving numerology (see above) and magical applications of sound.

Rolfing® (**structural integration, structural processing**): Deep-massage technique of "muscular realignment" promoted mainly for back and neck problems. Proponents also claim it facilitates weight loss, relieves anxiety, and increases stamina and self-esteem. Ida P. Rolf, Ph.D. (1896–1979), an organic chemist who had studied yoga and chiropractic, developed the method in New York in the 1930s. She compared her technique to "rebuilding a sagging or bulging brick wall, rather than trying to prop it up by artificial means." The Rolf Institute in Boulder, Colorado, founded in 1971, quotes her in a pamphlet: "Rolfers make a life study of relating bodies and their fields to the earth and its gravity field, and we so organize the body that the gravity field can reinforce the body's energy field." Rolfers adjust the massage when they supposedly detect areas of "energy imbalance" within the body. The standard rolfing series consists of ten sessions, each lasting from one hour to ninety minutes and costing between $60 and $100. Practitioners focus each session on a different body part. According to rolfing, the body may become rigid because of emotional trauma. Proponents claim that one's posture reveals past traumatic experiences, that rolfing effects emotional and "energetic" release, and that this alleged release restores the flow of "vital energy" and integrates mind and body (see Chapter 10).

Rubenfeld synergy method (Rubenfeld synergy): Form of body-oriented psychotherapy based partly on the Alexander technique (see above). Onetime orchestra conductor Ilana Rubenfeld developed the method in the early 1960s. A brochure describing a 1993 conference cosponsored by the Fetzer Institute (see Chapter 4) quotes her: "The body is the sacred sanctuary of the soul." According to a brochure from the Rubenfeld Center, in New York City, "emotions and memories stored in our beings often result in energy blocks, tensions, and imbalances." In a supplementary article, Rubenfeld states: "The body, mind, emotions, and spirit all form a dynamic and unitary—although not necessarily a unified—structure." Rubenfeld synergy involves aura analysis, "intentional and noninvasive" touch, kinesthesia, dreamwork (see above), and humor. Practitioners are called "synergists." (See Chapter 12.)

Schuessler (Schussler) biochemic system of medicine (biochemic system of medicine, biochemic medicine, tissue salts therapy): Quasi-homeopathic, naturopathic approach founded in the late nineteenth century by German physician Wilhelm Heinrich Schuessler (or Schussler). Schuessler held that disease was always due to a deficiency correctable with one or more of a dozen inorganic compounds called "cell salts" or "tissue salts": the fluoride, phosphate, and sulfate salts of calcium; the chloride, phosphate, and sulfate salts of sodium and potassium; the phosphate salts of iron and magnesium; and silicon dioxide. He proposed administering these salts in minuscule amounts to effect self-healing. *The Biochemic System of Medicine* (1991) quotes Schuessler: "The inorganic substances in the blood and tissues are sufficient to heal all diseases which are curable at all. The question whether this or that disease is or is not dependent on the existence of fungi, germs or bacilli is of no importance in biochemic treatment because this treatment goes to the basic cause of the trouble, and, by supplying to the cells the cell-salts needed for a normal condition to exist, thereby destroys the breeding place for the fungi, germs, or bacilli.... Chronic diseases can be cured by minute doses of cell-salts." In *The Complete Natural-Health Consultant* (1987), naturopath Michael van Straten wrote: "We now know that Schuessler's dosages were far too small to be effective." Yet he added that the "tissue salts" are "very beneficial" and may work by "giving a message to the body to absorb more of a certain substance or to get rid of it if there is an excess."

Sclerology: Practice of examining the sclera (white portion of the eye) for lines, discolorations, and other markings, purportedly to discover the condition of certain body organs.

Scrying (crystal gazing, crystal ball, crystalomancy): Looking at a candle flame, a transparent object, or something with a reflective surface (usually a globe of quartz glass) purportedly to learn about future events or to acquire occult knowledge. "Scry" is short for "descry"—"to see (something obscure)." Although proponents use the terms "scrying" and "crystal gazing" interchangeably, the former is the more general term. When a mirror is the object of scrying, the method is also called mirror-gazing. When water is its focus, the method is also called hydromancy.

Seichim: Purported ancient Egyptian healing art featuring *seichim* ("activating, ecstatic 'heart' energy"), the seichim "power mantra," and "goddess energy visualization."

Seichim reiki: Variant of seichim (see above) that purportedly involves accessing "interdimensional planes" and "empowering" crystals.

Seiki-jutsu: Japanese method wherein a "therapist" allegedly transfers "universal healing energy" (*seiki*) to a patient. The "transfer point" is the hair whorl at the crown of the patient's head. Some "therapists" place their hands on the patient's head and one of their knees against the sacrum.

Self-applied health enhancement methods (SAHEM): Variant of self-healing (see below) developed by acupuncturist Roger Jahnke. The methods fall into four categories: (1) gentle movements and postures—e.g., tai chi (see below), (2) self-massage—e.g., auricular reflexology (see above), (3) breathing exercises, and (4) relaxation practices.

Self-healing (direct healing): Alleged curing of oneself exclusively by tapping one's "innate healing potential" or "vital force" through affirmations and/or prayer. According to proponents, self-healing is sometimes instantaneous. George W. Meek described self-healing in *Healers and the Healing Process* (1977): "A healer does NOT do the healing. It is accomplished by his *reinforcing or supplementing the patient's own extraordinary capability of self-healing*. Each of the patient's basic systems . . . is an absolute marvel of perfection. The same level of perfection exists in all of the organs of the body. This fine physical body is the product of millions of years of development by the Creator."

Shamanism (shamanic healing, shamanistic medicine): Any indigenous magico-religious "healing" system whose core doctrine is that all healing involves a spirit world.

Shiatsu (shiatzu, schiatsu, shiatsu therapy): Japanese form of "therapeutic" massage in which practitioners apply pressure with the palms and four fingers of each hand to areas of the body relating to acupuncture. "Shiatsu" is the abbreviation of a Japanese word that literally means "finger-pressure treatment." The goal of shiatsu is to promote health by increasing the flow of *ki* in the body. It is based on both acupuncture theory and amma (see above). The major types of shiatsu are: (1) shiatsu massage, which is based largely on amma, (2) acupressure, a strictly manual variant of acupuncture, and (3) Zen shiatsu. The late Shizuto Masunaga developed Zen shiatsu. Unlike the two other major forms, it incorporates *kyo-jitsu*—the localizing of "imbalances" of *ki* by palpation (touch). In Zen shiatsu, practitioners apply less pressure than in shiatsu massage or acupressure (see Chapter 10).

Siddha (Siddha medicine): Tamil version of ayurveda. "Tamil" refers to a traditional culture of southern India and northern Sri Lanka. Siddha medicine emphasizes "remedies" containing minerals such as mercury, sulfur, and gold. "Siddha" is the Sanskrit word for "perfection."

Silva mind control (Silva mind control system, Silva method): Form of meditation developed by Texas-born electronics engineer José Silva. It is a variant of creative visualization (see above) and self-healing (see above), includes dreamwork (see above), and purportedly effects alpha rhythm—a pattern of electrical oscillations that occur in the brain when one is awake and relaxed. Proponents claim that the Silva method can facilitate weight loss, strengthen the immune system, foster extrasensory perception (ESP), and enable telepathy. In *The Alternative Health Guide* (1983), Brian Inglis and Ruth West stated: "The faculty for extrasensory perception, on which Silva places great emphasis, is worked on in particular to see if the students can project themselves to other places, or backward and forward in time."

Simonton method: Variant of creative visualization (see above) developed by radiation oncologist Oscar Carl Simonton, M.D., and his former wife, psychologist Stephanie Matthews-Simonton. Cancer patients following this method may visualize their white blood cells (representing the immune system) as dynamic, and their cancer cells as weak. The resource guide to "Healing and the Mind with Bill Moyers" (see Chapter 4) states that Dr. Simonton's "basic premise" is that "cancer is a message of love and an invitation to become who we truly are."

Six healing sounds: Sequence of vocalizations and postures. Performance of each sound/posture combination supposedly cools and cleanses an associated Chinese "organ." (See "Healing *tao*" above.)

Soaring crane Qigong (crane style *chi gong*): Simplified and allegedly fast-acting form of Qigong (see above) developed by Zhao Jin-Xiang. Shen Rong-er introduced it in the United States.

Sotai (sotai therapy, sotai treatment): Form of bodywork developed in Japan by Keizo Hashimoto, M.D. His illustrated handbook, *Sotai: Balance and Health Through Natural Movement* (1983), defines sotai as "a method enabling human beings to adapt to their environment by harmonizing respiration, ingestion, physical movements and mental activity." The word "sotai" is a combination of two Japanese characters meaning "work" (*so*) and "body" (*tai*)—"bodywork." Sotai purportedly uses the "liver meridian"—"one of the channels or pathways for the flow of vital energy in Oriental medicine." The book promotes Hashimoto's method for arthritis, the common cold, constipation, diarrhea, diabetes, edema of the hands, deteriorating eyesight, facial palsy, fatigue, hangovers, humpback, insomnia, liver cirrhosis, migraines, nasal obstructions, palpitations, scoliosis (abnormal curvature of the spine), shortness of breath, whiplash, "depression due to hypertension," and other health conditions. In the afterword, Japanese chiropractor Kenzo Kase states: "All disease is cured by the power of nature. God is the only one who can heal wounds; all man can do is bandage the wound."

Soul part integration: Adjunct to soul retrieval (see below). It is a form of "shamanic journeying" that supposedly reintegrates "soul parts" with the client's "vital life force."

Soul retrieval: Form of "spiritual healing" fostered by Sandra Ingerman. It involves "journeying" to "other realms" to regain "lost parts of the soul." Ingerman holds an M.A. degree in integral counseling psychology (a variant of transpersonal psychology) from the California Institute of Integral Studies in San Francisco. The school's 1988–1990 catalog stated that one of its objectives is "the integration of the religious, mythic and symbolic philosophies of ancient traditions with the empirical, analytic paradigms of modern science." Ingerman recommends soul retrieval for suicidal tendencies and for psychological problems due to abuse, rape, or trauma. (See "Transpersonal psychology" below.)

Spinal balancing: Variant of craniosacral balancing (see above) that focuses on the vertebrae.

Spirit healing (spiritual healing): Pseudotherapeutic form of channeling (see above) whose advocates ascribe healing to divine power or to doctors in the spirit world.

Spirit surgery: Imaginary surgery performed by otherworldly "healing entities" at the behest of a "spiritual healer."

Spiritual psychology: "Healing modality" based on anthroposophy, archetypal psychology, and Jungian psychology (see above for all). The Winter/ Spring 1994 catalog of the New York Open Center (see Chapter 10) states that the legend of the Holy Grail is a "guiding myth" of spiritual psychology and that its themes include "the destructiveness of spirit without soul" and "the suffering of soul in the absence of spirit."

Sufi healing: Tradition of faith healing (see above) based on Sufism, a multiform mystical tradition related to Islam that developed mainly in Persia (Iran). It is based particularly on the teachings of one of the largest Sufi orders, the Chishti order, which is eight hundred years old. Sufi "healers" function as guides to patient "self-diagnosis" by means of hypnosis. They chant prayers and pass their hands over the patient. Sufi healing also involves a dietetic system akin to that of ayurveda (see Chapter 5); a system of fasting that includes Ramadan, a month of total daytime abstention from food and water; herbal formulas; and a set of postures and associated Arabic sayings. Sufism categorizes foods and herbs according to their alleged "metabolic value": "hot" substances strengthen metabolism; "cold" substances lower it. Digestion supposedly gives rise to four "essences": blood essence (hot and moist), phlegm essence (cold and moist), bilious essence (hot and dry), and atrabilious essence (cold and dry). An "imbalance" of any "essence" purportedly leads to disease, and the first goal of Sufi "treatment" is to restore the alleged maladapted essence. In *The Book of Sufi Healing* (1991), abu-Abdullah Moinuddin, sheik of the American order of Chistis, states: "In addition to human souls and angels, Allah also created jinns. Whereas He created humans from the four elements of earth, water, air, and fire, He made the jinns from ' smokeless fire.' The jinns . . . can from time to time assume human form. . . . They have great effect upon human affairs and frequently cause imbalances that we would identify as disease. A prime example is colic in infants, who are especially prone to the influence of jinns. Certain herbal substances and recitations are used to dispel jinns."

Suggestive therapy (suggestive therapy work, suggestive therapeutics): Pseudotherapeutic phase of concept-therapy (see above and Chapter 13), based on the "power of suggestion." It is a variant of both *psi* healing (see above) and self-healing (see above). Suggestive therapy involves spinal "adjustments," "healing suggestions," a diet "to eliminate toxins," and food combining (see above).

Suggestive therapy zone procedure (zone therapy diagnosis, health zone analysis, concept-therapy adjusting technique, zone testing): Pseudodiagnostic phase of concept-therapy (see above and Chapter 13), based on a variant of chiropractic subluxation theory.

Synchronicity: "Acausal connecting principle"—the supposed equivalent of a cause—posited by Carl Jung (see above) to account for meaningful but apparently accidental concurrences or sequences of events. Jung held that his "synchronistic principle"—which he equated with the *tao* (see Chapter 6)— was the basis of both astrology and the "science" of the *I Ching* (see above).

Synergy hypnosis: Combination of hypnosis, neuro-linguistic programming (see above), "psychegenic" imagery, and "energy and breathing techniques." (See "Creative visualization" above.)

Systematic nutritional muscle testing (SNMT): Purportedly an extremely efficient and easy-to-master form of "muscle-testing" à la applied kinesiology (see above).

Tai chi (tai chi chuan, *tai ji*, *tai ji chuan*, *tai ji quan*): Ancient, yoga-like Chinese system of ballet-like exercises designed for health, self-defense, and spiritual development. "*Quan*" means "boxing." Tai chi was supposedly revealed in a dream to a Taoist sage. Extremely popular in modern China, the practice of tai chi supposedly facilitates the flow of *chi* through the body by dissolving blockages both within the body and between the body and the environment. Traditional tai chi prescribes about 108 to 128 postures, including repetitions. The difficulty lies in concatenating the postures into circular movements. In the Spring 1993 issue of *Qi: The Journal of Traditional Eastern Health & Fitness*, Chinese biologist Tang You-yue states that tai chi is the "integration" of Qigong and Chinese martial arts and that mastery of Qigong is a prerequisite for mastering tai chi.

Tantra: Yogic "sexual healing." (See Chapter 5.)

Taoist five element nutrition (Taoist healing diet): System of food combining based on astrology and the Chinese theory of "five elements." The term "five elements" derives from two Chinese words: *wu* ("five") and *xing* ("move" or "walk"). Its implicit meaning is "five processes." According to ancient Chinese tradition, earth, metal, water, wood, and fire are manifestations ("phases" or "transformations") of *chi* and compose everything. In Chinese medicine, each "element" symbolizes a category of related functions and qualities: "earth" represents balance or neutrality; "metal," a period of decline; "water," a state of maximum rest leading to a change of functional direction; "wood," a growth phase; and "fire," maximum activity. (See "Healing *tao*" above.)

Taoist Qigong (Daoist *chi kung*): Form of Qigong (see above) focused on the cultivation of morality, slowing the aging process, and rejuvenation. Practitioners also use Taoist Qigong for healing and to develop "internal power."

Tarot: Pack of playing cards (usually twenty-two, but sometimes seventy-eight) used in fortunetelling. The tarot consists of a joker and cards depicting vices, virtues, and "elemental forces." *Mysteries of Mind, Space and Time: The Unexplained* (1992) states: "Ideally, to make consulting the Tarot a true divinatory method, each practitioner should decide exactly what meaning to attach to each card—even if this departs widely from what is commonly held to be the meaning."

Telediagnosis (distant biological detection): Variant of pendular diagnosis (see above) wherein the practitioner holds a pendulum over a photo or drawing of the patient or over an object that has supposedly retained the patient's "radiation."

Theotherapy: Variant of self-healing (see above) developed by author Peter Lemesurier. According to this method, one determines—more or less unconsciously—which Greek god or goddess best symbolizes one's disease; then one treats the disease by trying to adopt the godly characteristics one considers positive and sustainable. Theotherapy holds that every divine characteristic is a therapy and that every symptom is a healing tool.

Therapeutic eurythmy (therapeutic eurhythmy, curative eurhythmy, curative eurythmy): Pseudomedical form of eurythmy—so-called visible speech, visible song, or sacred dance. It supposedly contributes to the restoration of a proper flow of "astral energies." Eurythmy (also called eurythmics) is an anthroposophical method. It holds that linguistic sounds have counterparts in postures and movements involving mainly the arms and hands (see "Anthroposophical medicine" above).

Therapeutic touch (TT): "A method (derived from the laying-on of hands) of using the hands to direct human energies to help or heal someone who is ill," as defined by Dolores Krieger, Ph.D., R.N., in *The Therapeutic Touch: How to Use Your Hands to Help or to Heal* (1986). Therein, Krieger ascribed her interest in the laying on of hands largely to Dora Kunz, who was "born with a unique ability to perceive subtle energies around living beings" and studied under occultist Charles W. Leadbeater. Krieger and Kunz developed TT in the early 1970s, and the first center for TT was established in a Catholic-oriented school of nursing. In her book, Krieger urged students of her method to record their dreams, consult the *I Ching*, and draw mandalas—aids to meditation symbolizing the unity of the soul with the universe. In the Winter 1993 issue of *Skeptical Inquirer*, Professors Vern L. Bullough and Bonnie Bullough write: "The problem in doing research on TT is to demonstrate that real energy passes between therapist and patient, which no one has been able to do. Certainly any reduction in tension [resulting from TT] is likely to reduce pain . . . but this could also be done by watching a comedy on television or tapes of old movies." Noncontact therapeutic touch is a form of TT in which the practitioner does not touch the patient.

Tibetan medicine (*Emchi*): System akin to ayurveda (see Chapter 5), positing the same physiological forces (*pitta, kapha*, and *vata*) and involving gods, evil spirits, and fate.

Tibetan pulsing (Tibetan pulsing healing): Ancient oriental "art" involving bodywork and "eye-reading." Practitioners ascribe disease to specific organs by means of "eye reading." According to Tibetan pulsing, "bio-electrical energy" travels along the bones of the human skeleton. Manual and vocal stimulation of specific areas of the skin ("pulse points") and the use of colors associated with specific organs allegedly dissolve blockages in the nervous system and free "life energy."

Toning: Vocal method originated by Laurel Keyes alleged to promote healing, creativity, and vitality. Toning supposedly enables "tuning in" to the "higher self," activates dormant "creative energy," brings new "life energy" to "inhibited" or "unbalanced" parts of the body, and cleanses the "whole being." It involves standing with eyes closed, relaxing the jaws, and expressing feelings by means of vocal sounds. Meditation and yogic postures sometimes accompany toning.

Touch for Health: System of energy balancing (see above) developed by chiropractor John F. Thie; a combination of applied kinesiology (see above) and "acupressure touch"—a gentle form of acupressure (see above). In *Touch for Health*, written with Mary Marks, Thie stated that the goal of chiropractic is to remove interferences between "innate intelligence," which allegedly runs the body, and "universal intelligence," which allegedly runs the world.

Trager (the Trager approach, Tragerwork, Tragering, Trager psychophysical integration®): Form of bodywork developed by Milton Trager, M.D., a former boxer and acrobat. In the 1940s, Trager obtained a "Doctorate of Physical Medicine" from the L.A. College of Drugless Physicians. According to *The Encyclopedia of Alternative Health Care* (1989), after seventy American medical schools had rejected him, Trager earned his M.D. degree at a Mexican university. In 1958, he became one of the first eight initiates of the Maharishi Mahesh Yogi in the United States (see Chapter 5). Practitioners supposedly work in a meditative state termed "hook-up" (see "Trager mentastics" below). The *Family Guide to Natural Medicine: How to Stay Healthy the Natural Way* (1993) states: "During a typical session, the practitioner gently and rhythmically rocks, cradles, and moves the client's body so as to encourage the client to see that freedom of movement and relaxation are entirely possible. The aim of the treatment is not to manipulate or massage specific joints, but to promote a feeling of lightness, limberness, and well-being." Proponents recommend the Trager approach for asthma, autism, chronic back pain, emphysema, multiple sclerosis, muscular dystrophy, polio, sciatica, and other conditions.

Trager mentastics (mentastics®): System of body movements developed by Milton Trager, M.D. (see above), and described in his book *Trager Mentastics: Movement as a Way to Agelessness*. Trager defined "mentastics" as "mental gymnastics"—"mentally directed movements that suggest to the mind feelings of lightness, freedom, openness, grace and pleasure resulting in an ageless body." He claimed that mentastics could reverse the aging process. The system's "most basic and important ingredient" is "hook-up"—a "meditative process" and perfect "natural state of being" wherein one supposedly connects with a measurable, transpersonal, life-giving, regulatory force.

Transcendental meditation (TM): Form of meditation developed by the Maharishi Mahesh Yogi. It involves sitting in a comfortable position with one's eyes closed for fifteen to twenty minutes in the morning and evening. Meditators silently repeat a mantra—a "secret" magic word that a TM teacher supposedly chooses expressly for the initiate. (See Chapter 5.)

"Transformation" program: One of psychotherapist Dr. Wayne W. Dyer's audiocassette programs for self-development. The program is subtitled: "You'll See It When You Believe It." (See "'Awakened Life' program" above.)

Transformational bodywork: Combination of aura balancing (see above), chakra healing (see above), reiki (see above), and "integrative body work."

Transpersonal psychology (transpersonal counseling): Combination of Jungian psychology, psychosynthesis, and Eastern mysticism emphasizing self-transcendence, meditation, and prayer. In 1917, Carl Jung apparently was the first to use the word "transpersonal" (*üeberpersönlich*). Psychiatrist Stanislav

Grof (see "Holotropic breathwork" above) coined the term "transpersonal psychology." (See "Jungian psychology" and "Psychosynthesis" above.)

Triggers™ mind programming system (triggers): Audiocassette "course" developed by hypnotist and certified social worker Stanley Mann, author of *Triggers: The Technology of Super-Motivation*. Zygon International in Redmond, Washington, markets the program. Zygon suggests that "triggers" is the "Holy Grail of self-improvement" and enables users to harness their "magic powers" and "heal illness with a mere thought." Zygon also claims that the system enables users to experience the power of their "various inner selves" and "instantly motivates" them to attract money, become persuasive leaders, end procrastination, erase fears, improve golf scores, improve their love life, lose weight, master new skills immediately, quit smoking, solve any problem, and unleash "secret wisdom."

***Tui na* (*tui na an mo*):** Form of Chinese Qigong massage involving a wide variety of hand movements. "*Tui*" means "push"; "*na*" means "grab"; and "*an mo*" means "massage." Proponents recommend it primarily for external injuries.

Twelve steps: Theistic system that purportedly advances recovery from various addictions and compulsive behaviors. Twelve-step programs oblige participants to foster a connection with God or an alleged transpersonal "spiritual energy" or superhuman "power." Their supposed goal is the integration of body, mind, and spirit. In *Codependents' Guide to the Twelve Steps* (1992), Melody Beattie states: "God is fundamental to recovery and fundamental to the psychic and soul-level change and healing we're seeking.... Struggle with the Higher Power concept. Struggle all you need to.... Struggle until you find your Higher Power and know your God cares about the largest and most minute details of your life." According to *The Twelve Steps to Happiness: A Handbook for All Twelve Steppers* (1990), the third step suggests that followers turn over their "very existence" to God—"that unknown and possibly nonexistent Power"; the eleventh step is that in which followers become sure of God's existence; and the twelfth step directs followers to spread the "message" of the twelve steps. There are more than a dozen twelve-step organizations, including Alcoholics Anonymous, Emotions Anonymous, Fundamentalists Anonymous, Overeaters Anonymous, and Sexaholics Anonymous. The phrasing of the twelve steps varies according to the particular organization.

Unani (Unani medicine): Islamic combination of ancient Greek medicine and ayurveda. It posits four basic "elements"—earth, fire, water, and air—and four humors—phlegm, blood, yellow bile (choler), and black bile. The goal of Unani is the "balancing" of these humors. Temperament supposedly stems from the dominant humor and is the basis of "diagnosis" and treatment. For example, anger and irritability allegedly manifest an excess of yellow bile. "Unani" is the Arabic word for "Greek." (See Chapter 5.)

Urine therapy (uropathy, auto-urine-therapy, *amaroli, shivambu kalpa*): "Remedy" with Indian roots wherein the patient's urine is ingested, injected, introduced into the rectum, and/or used topically (see Chapter 5).

Vita flex (reflex system): Variant of reflexology (see above) developed by Stanley Burroughs, author of *Healing for the Age of Enlightenment* (1976). Vita flex is one of the three major components of his theistic system of "natural healing." The other major components are color therapy and the lemonade diet (see above for both). In the fourth edition of his book, Burroughs claimed that the human body has more than five thousand "Vita Flex points of control." He proposed a last-ditch mode of vita flex with four variations in which the practitioner: (1) treats the affected part of the patient's body by applying pressure to the same part of the practitioner's body, (2) uses the manual technique on a third party (a stand-in), (3) visualizes treating the affected part of the patient, or (4) visualizes the patient effecting self-healing (see above). Burroughs declared: "Medicine is a form of fiction that feeds on ignorance of the true needs of the body to restore normal health and retain it."

Viviano method: Approach to behavior modification developed by Ann Viviano, a New York psychologist, minister, reiki master, and practitioner of neuro-linguistic programming (see above). It purportedly uses principles of psychology, modern medicine, quantum physics, New Age mysticism, and meditation.

Warriorobics: Blend of aerobics, aikido (see above), and *ki* breathing (see above) developed by Henry Smith.

White tantra: Alleged precursor of hatha yoga (see above) involving postures, *pranayama* (breathing exercises), and meditation. The practice supposedly balances the body's positive and negative "energies" and the brain's "two sides." (See Chapter 5.)

Whole person bodywork: Form of aura balancing and chakra healing (see above for both).

Wise woman healing (wisewoman healing ways, wisewoman ways): Feminine variant of nature cure (see above) involving medical herbalism, meditation, and ritual. Wise woman healing stresses empiricism and intuition. It is based partly on the notion that the moon guides women's bodies.

Witchcraft: Generally, the use of amulets (or talismans), magical "potions," magical rituals, and/or spells. For example, *The Complete Book of Magic and Witchcraft* (1980) describes a "cure" for jaundice: "12 large earthworms, baked on a shovel and ground to powder, drunk in potion." The author, Kathryn Paulsen, added parenthetically: "Somewhat poisonous effects have been noticed from this recipe." For madness, she recommended consuming a drink containing mild honey and salt—before sunrise and from a seashell; and for strength, a black spider between two slices of buttered bread.

Yantra yoga (Tibetan yantra yoga): Tibetan Buddhist variant of hatha yoga (see above). It emphasizes continuous movement. (See Chapter 5.)

Yoga: An ancient philosophy whose goal is the liberation of the "true self" from material bonds via silencing of the mind. It features meditation, postures, and breathing exercises. Many schools of yoga are described on pages 54–56 and throughout this glossary.

Yoga of perfect sight: System of exercises for treating visual dysfunctions, promoted by a Dr. R.S. Agarwal.

Yoga therapy: "Psychotherapeutic" variant of hatha yoga (see above) based on the notion that disease is the cumulative lodging of "undigested experiences" in the "body/mind."

Zarlen therapy: "Mental healing" technique "discovered" in 1984 by Jonathan Sherwood in New Zealand. It supposedly affords users access to knowledge acquired during previous incarnations. "Zarlen" is the name of Sherwood's alleged spirit guide. According to the Queensland Awareness Center in Queensland, Australia, "When Zarlen first made contact with Jonathan in 1984, he stated that he had not had communication with humans for over 25,000 years and that he had returned to assist with a spiritual transition which the human race was about to pass through." Proponents recommend Zarlen therapy for numerous ailments, including brain damage, colorblindness, dyslexia, and varicose veins.

Zen Alexander technique: "Interdisciplinary" approach involving the Alexander technique (see above) and "Chinese energetic synthesis of MindBodySoulSpirit." It allegedly cultivates "unique synergistic healing powers" with which one can create one's own reality.

Zen-touch™: Purportedly powerful and painless variant of shiatsu promoted by the School of Healing Arts in San Diego, California.

Zone therapy (reflex zone therapy): Early form of Western reflexology (see above) introduced in the United States in 1913 by William H. Fitzgerald, M.D., a specialist in diseases of the ear, nose, and throat. Fitzgerald divided the human body into ten zones and taught that "bioelectrical" energy flowed through these zones to "reflex points" in the hands and feet. His method, which was also called zonotherapy, involved the fastening of wire springs around toes. Today, zone therapy may include the attachment of clothespins to fingertips and the use of pencils and aluminum combs. Fitzgerald's associate, Edwin F. Bowers, M.D., coined the term "zone therapy." (See Chapter 10.)

Bibliography

This is a partial list of books and articles that have contributed to my understanding of mystical "healing" and supernaturalism. I have marked some of the books that I found especially useful or interesting with an asterisk.

Critical Literature—"Alternative" Healthcare and Related Beliefs

G.O. Abell and B. Singer (editors). *Science and the Paranormal: Probing the Existence of the Supernatural.* New York: Charles Scribner's Sons, 1983.

*S. Barrett and W.T. Jarvis (editors). *The Health Robbers: A Close Look at Quackery in America.* Buffalo, N.Y.: Prometheus Books, 1993.

R.J. Brenneman. *Deadly Blessings: Faith Healing on Trial.* Buffalo, N.Y.: Prometheus Books, 1990.

*K. Butler. *A Consumer's Guide to "Alternative Medicine": A Close Look at Homeopathy, Acupuncture, Faith-Healing, and Other Unconventional Treatments.* Buffalo, N.Y.: Prometheus Books, 1992.

R. Ernst. *Weakness Is a Crime: The Life of Bernarr Macfadden.* Syracuse, N.Y.: Syracuse University Press, 1991.

M. Fishbein. *Fads and Quackery in Healing.* New York: Blue Ribbon Books, Inc., 1932.

K. Frazier (ed.). *The Hundredth Monkey and Other Paradigms of the Paranormal: A Skeptical Inquirer Collection.* Buffalo, N.Y.: Prometheus Books, 1991

_____ *Science Confronts the Paranormal.* Buffalo, N.Y.: Prometheus Books, 1986.

*R.C. Fuller. *Alternative Medicine and American Religious Life.* New York: Oxford University Press, 1989.

H. Gordon. *Channeling into the New Age: The "Teachings" of Shirley MacLaine and Other Such Gurus.* Buffalo, N.Y.: Prometheus Books, 1988.

T. Hines. *Pseudoscience and the Paranormal: A Critical Examination of the Evidence.* Buffalo, N.Y.: Prometheus Books, 1988.

L.E. Jerome. *Crystal Power: The Ultimate Placebo Effect.* Buffalo, N.Y.: Prometheus Books, 1989.

J. Money. *The Destroying Angel: Sex, Fitness and Food in the Legacy of Degeneracy Theory, Graham Crackers, Kellogg's Corn Flakes and American Health History.* Buffalo, N.Y.: Prometheus Books, 1985.

J. Randi. *The Faith Healers.* Buffalo, N.Y.: Prometheus Books, 1989.

_____ *Flim-Flam! Psychics, ESP, Unicorns and Other Delusions.* Buffalo, N.Y.: Prometheus Books, 1982.

J. Raso. *Mystical Diets: Paranormal, Spiritual, and Occult Nutrition Practices.* Buffalo, N.Y.: Prometheus Books, 1993.

J.A. Roth with R.R. Hanson. *Health Purifiers and Their Enemies: A Study of the Natural Health Movement in the United States with a Comparison to Its Counterpart in Germany.* New York: Prodist, 1977.

*D. Stalker and C. Glymour. *Examining Holistic Medicine.* Buffalo, N.Y.: Prometheus Books, 1989.

R.L. Taylor. *Health Fact, Health Fiction: Getting through the Media Maze.* Dallas, Tex.: Taylor Publishing Co., 1990.

*J.F. Zwicky, A.F. Hafner, S. Barrett, and W.T. Jarvis. *Reader's Guide to "Alternative" Health Methods.* Chicago: American Medical Association, 1993.

Christian Literature Critical of "Alternative" Healthcare and Related Beliefs

*J. Ankerberg and J. Weldon. *Can You Trust Your Doctor? The Complete Guide to New Age Medicine and Its Threat to Your Family.* Brentwood, Tenn.: Wolgemuth and Hyatt, 1991.

R. Chandler. *Understanding the New Age.* Dallas: Word Publishing, 1988.

D. Groothuis. *Confronting the New Age: How to Resist a Growing Religious Movement.* Downers Grove, Ill.: InterVarsity Press, 1988.

Critical Literature—Mysticism, Occultism, and Religion

*R. Basil (ed.). *Not Necessarily the New Age: Critical Essays.* Buffalo, N.Y.: Prometheus Books, 1988.

E. Becker. *The Denial of Death.* New York: Macmillan, 1973.

E. Carlson. *The Phantoms of Divinity.* Buffalo, N.Y.: Prometheus Books, 1992.

E. Clark. The price of faith. *Yankee*, July 1992. (A comprehensive review of Christian Science.)

T.S. Clements. *Science vs. Religion*. Buffalo, N.Y.: Prometheus Books, 1990.

*W. Harwood. *Mythology's Last Gods: Yahweh and Jesus*. Buffalo, N.Y.: Prometheus Books, 1992.

S. Hassan. *Combatting Cult Mind Control*. Rochester, Vt.: Park Street Press, 1990.

B.C. Johnson. *The Atheist Debater's Handbook*. Buffalo, N.Y.: Prometheus Books, 1983.

*P. Kurtz. *The Transcendental Temptation: A Critique of Religion and the Paranormal*. Buffalo, N.Y.: Prometheus Books, 1991.

*G.A. Larue. *The Supernatural, the Occult and the Bible*. Buffalo, N.Y.: Prometheus Books, 1990.

*D. Radner and M. Radner. *Science and Unreason*. Belmont, Cal.: Wadsworth Publishing Co., 1982.

*B. Russell. *Religion and Science*. New York: Oxford University Press, 1961.

* _____ *Why I Am Not a Christian and Other Essays on Religion and Related Subjects*. New York: Simon & Schuster, 1957.

*T. Schultz (ed.). *The Fringes of Reason: A Whole Earth Catalog*. New York: Crown Publishers, 1989.

*J.F. Schumaker. *Wings of Illusion: The Origin, Nature and Future of Paranormal Belief*. Buffalo, N.Y.: Prometheus Books, 1990.

A. Seckel (ed.). *Bertrand Russell on God and Religion*. Buffalo, N.Y.: Prometheus Books, 1986.

D. Sklar. *The Nazis and the Occult*. New York: Dorset Press, 1989.

*G.H. Smith. *Atheism: The Case Against God*. Buffalo, N.Y.: Prometheus Books, 1989.

V.J. Stenger. *Physics and Psychics: The Search for a World Beyond the Senses*. Buffalo, N.Y.: Prometheus Books, 1990.

J. Webb. *The Occult Establishment*. La Salle, Ill.: Open Court, 1985.

_____ *The Occult Underground*. La Salle, Ill.: Open Court, 1974.

Proponent Literature—"Alternative" Healthcare

H.E. Altenberg. *Holistic Medicine: A Meeting of East and West*. New York: Japan Publications, Inc., 1992.

D. Black: *Health at the Crossroads: Exploring the Conflict Between Natural Healing and Conventional Medicine*. Springville, Ut.: Tapestry Press, 1988.

M. Bricklin. *The Practical Encyclopedia of Natural Healing*. New York: MJF Books, 1983.

M. Coddington. *Seekers of the Healing Energy: Reich, Cayce, the Kahunas, and Other Masters of the Vital Force*. Rochester, Vt.: Healing Arts Press, 1990.

*H. Day. *Encyclopaedia of Natural Health and Healing*. Santa Barbara, Cal.: Woodbridge Press Publishing Co., 1979.

B.M. Dossey, L. Keegan, L.G. Kolkmeier, and C. E. Guzzetta. *Holistic Health Promotion: A Guide for Practice.* Rockville, Md.: Aspen Publishers, 1989.

L. Dossey. *Space, Time, and Medicine.* Boston: Shambhala Publications, 1985.

*N. Drury. *The Healing Power: A Handbook of Alternative Medicine and Natural Health.* London: Frederick Muller Ltd., 1981.

R. Grossinger. *Planet Medicine: From Stone Age Shamanism to Post-Industrial Healing.* Berkeley, Cal.: North Atlantic Books, 1987.

A.E. Guinness (ed.). *Family Guide to Natural Medicine: How to Stay Healthy the Natural Way.* Pleasantville, N.Y.: Reader's Digest Association, 1993.

B.Q. Hafen and K.J. Frandsen. *From Acupuncture to Yoga: Alternative Methods of Healing.* Englewood Cliffs, N.J.: Prentice-Hall, 1983.

H. Holzer. *Beyond Medicine: The Facts about Unorthodox Treatments and Psychic Healing.* New York: Ballantine Books, 1987.

B. Inglis. *Fringe Medicine.* London: Faber and Faber, 1964.

*_____ *Natural Medicine.* Glasgow, Great Britain: William Collins Sons and Co. Ltd., 1980.

T. Kaptchuk and M. Croucher. *The Healing Arts: Exploring the Medical Ways of the World.* New York: Summit Books, 1987.

D. Kunz (ed.). *Spiritual Aspects of the Healing Arts.* Wheaton, Ill.: Theosophical Publishing House, 1985.

B.M. Ley. *Health Talks: Exclusive Interviews with Some of the Nation's Leading Authorities in Alternative Practices in Health and Nutrition.* Fargo, N.D.: Christopher Lawrence Communications, 1989.

B. McNeill and C. Guion (editors). *Noetic Sciences Collection 1980-1990: Ten Years of Consciousness Research.* Sausalito, Cal.: Institute of Noetic Sciences, 1991.

T. Monte and the editors of *EastWest Natural Health. World Medicine: The East West Guide to Healing Your Body.* New York: Jeremy P. Tarcher/Perigee Books, 1993.

Mysteries of the Unknown: Powers of Healing. Alexandria, Va.: Time-Life Books.

K.G. Olsen. *The Encyclopedia of Alternative Health Care.* New York: Simon & Schuster, 1989.

P. Pietroni. *The Greening of Medicine.* London: Victor Gollancz Ltd., 1991.

D.S. Rogo. *New Techniques of Inner Healing: Conversations with Contemporary Masters of Alternative Healing.* New York: Paragon House, 1992.

C.N. Shealy with A.S. Freese. *Occult Medicine Can Save Your Life: A Modern Doctor Looks at Unconventional Healing.* Columbus, O.: Brindabella Books, 1985.

M. Starck. *The Complete Handbook of Natural Healing.* St. Paul, Minn.: Llewellyn Publications, 1991.

M. van Straten. *The Complete Natural-Health Consultant: A Practical Handbook of Alternative Health Treatments.* New York: Simon & Schuster, 1987.

*A. Weil. *Health and Healing: Understanding Conventional and Alternative Medicine.* Boston: Houghton Mifflin, 1983.

M. Wood. *The Magical Staff: The Vitalist Tradition in Western Medicine.* Berkeley, Cal.: North Atlantic Books, 1992.

Proponent Literature—Mysticism, Occultism, and/or Religion

Anon. *Coming Back: The Science of Reincarnation.* Los Angeles: Bhaktivedanta Book Trust, 1982.

F. Capra. *The Tao of Physics: An Exploration of the Parallels Between Modern Physics and Eastern Mysticism. Second Edition.* New York: Bantam Books, 1984.

*M. Corner. *Does God Exist?* New York: St. Martin's Press, 1991.

L.A. Davis. *Toward a World Religion for the New Age.* Farmington, N.Y.: Coleman Publishing, 1983.

G. Doore. *What Survives? Contemporary Explorations of Life After Death.* Los Angeles: Jeremy P. Tarcher, Inc., 1990.

M. Ferguson. *The Aquarian Conspiracy: Personal and Social Transformation in Our Time.* Los Angeles: Jeremy P. Tarcher, Inc., 1987.

Joel. *Naked Through the Gate: A Spiritual Autobiography.* Eugene, Ore.: Center for Sacred Sciences, 1985.

H. Kung. *Does God Exist? An Answer for Today.* New York: Random House, 1981.

R.M. Lewis. *Mental Alchemy.* San Jose, Cal.: Supreme Grand Lodge of AMORC, Inc., 1984.

F.D. Peat. *Synchronicity: The Bridge Between Matter and Mind.* New York: Bantam Books, 1987.

Sri Swami Rama, V.V. Merchant, G. Wangyal, M. Chitrabhanu, and B. Singh. *Inner Paths.* Honesdale, Pa.: Himalayan International Institute of Yoga Science and Philosophy, 1979.

S. Rosen. *Food for the Spirit: Vegetarianism and the World Religions.* New York: Bala Books, 1987.

F.H. Ross and T. Hills. *The Great Religions by which Men Live.* New York: Ballantine Books, 1983.

D.W. Shriver, Jr. (ed.). *Medicine and Religion: Strategies of Care.* Pittsburgh: University of Pittsburgh Press, 1980.

H. Smith. *Beyond the Post-Modern Mind.* Wheaton, Ill.: Theosophical Publishing House, 1989.

_____ *The Religions of Man.* New York: Harper & Row, 1965.

J.M. Templeton and R.L. Herrmann. *The God Who Would Be Known: Revelations of the Divine in Contemporary Science.* San Francisco: Harper & Row, 1989.

P. Tillich. *The Meaning of Health: The Relation of Religion and Health.* Richmond, Cal.: North Atlantic Books, 1981.

E. Underhill. *Mysticism: A Study in the Nature and Development of Man's Spiritual Consciousness.* New York: Penguin Books, 1974.

G. Zukav. *The Dancing Wu-Li Masters: An Overview of the New Physics.* New York: Bantam Books, 1980.

_____ *The Seat of the Soul.* New York: Simon & Schuster, 1990.

Proponent Literature—Specific Systems, Methods, and Gurus

Actualism

R. Metzner. *Maps of Consciousness*. New York: Macmillan, 1971.

Acupuncture

F.F. Kao with J.J. Kao. *Acupuncture Therapeutics: An Introductory Text*. New Haven, Ct.: Eastern Press, 1973.

P. Marcus. *Acupuncture: A Patient's Guide*. New York: Thorsons Publishers Inc., 1985.

African holistic health

T.D. O'Neal. Holistic health: Outdated practices or a prescription for the future. *Upscale*, February/March 1991, pp. 72–74.

Alexander technique

F.M. Alexander. *The Alexander Technique: The Essential Writings of F. Matthias Alexander*. New York: Carol Publishing Group, 1990.

F.P. Jones. *Body Awareness in Action: A Study of the Alexander Technique*. New York: Schocken Books, 1979.

Alternative twelve steps

M. Cleveland and A.G. What does it mean to "work the steps"? *Changes*, February 1992, p. 46.

Angelic healing

J.M. Howard. *Commune with the Angels: A Heavenly Handbook*. Virginia Beach, Va.: A.R.E. Press, 1992.

Anthroposophy

V. Bott. *Anthroposophical Medicine: Spiritual Science and the Art of Healing*. Rochester, Vt.: Healing Arts Press, 1984.

S.E. Easton. *Man and World in the Light of Anthroposophy*. Hudson, N.Y.: Anthroposophic Press, 1989.

F.X. King. *Rudolf Steiner and Holistic Medicine: An Introduction to the Revolutionary Ideas of the Founder of Anthroposophy*. York Beach, Me.: Nicolas-Hays, Inc., 1987.

G. Schmidt. *Cancer and Nutrition*. Spring Valley, N.Y.: Anthroposophic Press, 1986.

_____ *The Dynamics of Nutrition: The Impulse of Rudolf Steiner's Spiritual Science for a New Nutritional Hygiene*. Wyoming, R.I.: Bio-Dynamic Literature, 1980.

_____ *The Essentials of Nutrition*. Wyoming, R.I.: Bio-Dynamic Literature, 1987.

R. Steiner. *Nutrition and Health: Two Lectures to Workmen*. Hudson, N.Y.: Anthroposophic Press, 1987.

_____ *The Universal Human: The Evolution of Individuality*. Hudson, N.Y.: Anthroposophic Press, Inc., 1990.

R. Steiner and I. Wegman. *Fundamentals of Therapy: An Extension of the Art of Healing through Spiritual Knowledge*. London: Rudolf Steiner Press, 1983.

Applied kinesiology
T. Valentine and C. Valentine with D.P. Hetrick. *Applied Kinesiology: Muscle Response in Diagnosis, Therapy and Preventive Medicine*. Rochester, Vt.: Healing Arts Press, 1987.

Aromatherapy
V.A. Worwood. *The Complete Book of Essential Oils and Aromatherapy*. San Rafael, Cal.: New World Library, 1991.

Auric massage technique
J.M. Howard. *Commune with the Angels: A Heavenly Handbook*. Virginia Beach, Va.: A.R.E. Press, 1992.

Ayurveda
R. Ballentine. *Diet and Nutrition: A Holistic Approach*. Honesdale, Pa.: Himalayan International Institute of Yoga Science and Philosophy of the U.S.A., 1982.
D. Chopra. *Ageless Body, Timeless Mind: The Quantum Alternative to Growing Old*. New York: Crown Publishers, 1993.
_____ *Creating Health: How to Wake Up the Body's Intelligence*. Boston: Houghton Mifflin, 1991.
_____ *Perfect Health: The Complete Mind/Body Guide*. New York: Crown Publishers, 1990.
_____ *Quantum Healing: Exploring the Frontiers of Mind/Body Medicine*. New York: Bantam Books, 1990.
_____ *Return of the Rishi: A Doctor's Story of Spiritual Transformation and Ayurvedic Healing*. Boston: Houghton Mifflin, 1991.
_____ *Unconditional Life: Mastering the Forces that Shape Personal Reality*. New York: Bantam Books, 1991.
V.B. Dash. *Fundamentals of Ayurvedic Medicine*. Seventh Revised Edition. Delhi, India: Konark Publishers Pvt. Ltd., 1989.
T.L. Devaraj. *Ayurveda for Healthy Living*. New Delhi, India: UBS Publishers' Distributors Ltd., 1992.
B. Heyn. *Ayurveda: The Indian Art of Natural Medicine and Life Extension*. Rochester, Vt.: Healing Arts Press, 1990.
V. Lad. *Ayurveda: The Science of Self-Healing. A Practical Guide*. Wilmot, Wis.: Lotus Light, 1985.
B.L. Raina. *Health Science in Ancient India*. New Delhi, India: Commonwealth Publishers, 1990.
Swami Rama. *A Practical Guide to Holistic Health*. Revised Edition. Honesdale, Pa.: Himalayan International Institute of Yoga Science and Philosophy, 1980.
R.E. Svoboda. *Ayurveda: Life, Health and Longevity*. New York: Penguin Books, 1992.
_____ *Prakruti: Your Ayurvedic Constitution*. Albuquerque, N.M.: Geocom Ltd., 1988.
S. Treadway and L. Treadway. *Ayurveda and Immortality*. Berkeley, Cal.: Celestial Arts, 1986.

Baby B.E.S.T.
M.T. Morter. *Baby B.E.S.T.: Infant Adjusting/Care.* Rogers, Ark.: Morter HealthSystem, 1991.

Bach flower therapy
E. Bach. *Heal Thyself: An Explanation of the Real Cause and Cure of Disease.* Saffron Walden, Essex, England: C.W. Daniel Co. Ltd., 1931.
T.W.H. Jones. *Dictionary of the Bach Flower Remedies: Positive and Negative Aspects.* Saffron Walden, Essex, England: C.W. Daniel Co. Ltd., 1984.

Baguazhang (circle walking)
D. Miller. Circle walking of baguazhang. *Qi: The Journal of Traditional Eastern Health & Fitness,* Vol. 3, No. 2, Summer 1993, pp. 34–39.

Bio energetic synchronization technique (B.E.S.T.)
M.T. Morter. *B.E.S.T.* Rogers, Ark.: Morter HealthSystem, 1980.

Bioenergetics
A. Lowen. *Bioenergetics.* New York: Penguin Books, 1976.

Bodymind centering
G. Hendricks and K. Hendricks. *Radiance! Breathwork, Movement and Body-Centered Psychotherapy.* Berkeley, Cal.: Wingbow Press, 1991.

Bodywork
J. Feltman (ed.). *Hands-On Healing: Massage Remedies for Hundreds of Health Problems.* Emmaus, Pa.: Rodale Press, 1989.
D.B. Lawrence. *Massage Techniques.* New York: Putnam Publishing Group, 1986.
F.M. Tappan. *Healing Massage Techniques: Holistic, Classic, and Emerging Methods. Second Edition.* Norwalk, Ct.: Appleton & Lange, 1988.

Bodywork tantra
H. Dull. *Bodywork Tantra on Land and in Water.* Middletown, Cal.: Harbin Springs Publishing, 1987.

Cayce, Edgar
B. Bolton. *Edgar Cayce Speaks.* New York: Avon Books, 1969.
H.H. Bro. *A Seer Out of Season: The Life of Edgar Cayce.* New York: Penguin Books, 1989.
*E.E. Cayce and H.L. Cayce. *The Outer Limits of Edgar Cayce's Power.* Virginia Beach. Va.: A.R.E. Press, 1971.
H.L. Cayce. *Venture Inward.* New York: Harper & Row, 1964.
W.A. McGarey. *The Edgar Cayce Remedies.* New York: Bantam Books, 1983.
W.A. McGarey et. al. *Physician's Reference Notebook.* Virginia Beach, Va.: A.R.E. Press, 1983.
A. Read, C. Ilstrup, and M. Gammon. *Edgar Cayce on Diet and Health.* New York: Warner Books, 1969.

H.J. Reilly and R.H. Brod. *The Edgar Cayce Handbook for Health Through Drugless Therapy*. New York: Macmillan, 1975.

J. Stearn. *Edgar Cayce—The Sleeping Prophet*. New York: Bantam Books, 1968.

T. Sugrue. *There Is a River: The Story of Edgar Cayce. Revised Edition*. Virginia Beach, Va.: A.R.E. Press, 1945.

Chinese health balls

H. Höting. *Chinese Health Balls: Practical Exercises*. Diever, Holland: Binkey Kok Publications, 1990.

Channeling

S. MacLaine. *Out on a Limb*. New York: Bantam Books, 1984.

Chinese medicine

R.M. Chin. *The Energy Within: The Science Behind Every Oriental Therapy from Acupuncture to Yoga*. New York: Paragon House, 1992.

*D. Eisenberg with T.L. Wright. *Encounters with Qi: Exploring Chinese Medicine*. New York: Viking Penguin, 1987.

T.J. Kaptchuk. *The Web That Has No Weaver: Understanding Chinese Medicine*. New York: Congdon & Weed, Inc., 1983.

Chinese Qigong massage

*J. Yang. *Chinese Qigong Massage: General Massage*. Jamaica Plain, Mass.: Yang's Martial Arts Association, 1992.

Chinese system of food cures

H.C. Lu. *Chinese System of Food Cures: Prevention and Remedies*. New York: Sterling Publishing Co., Inc., 1986.

Chiropractic

M. Bach. *The Chiropractic Story*. Austell, Ga.: Si-Nel Publishing & Sales Co., 1968.

T. McClusky and J. Dintenfass. *Your Health and Chiropractic. Revised Edition*. New York: Pyramid Books, 1962.

L. Sportelli. *Introduction to Chiropractic: A Natural Method of Health Care. Ninth Edition*. Palmerton, Pa.: Practice Makers Products, Inc., 1988.

C.A. Wilk. *Chiropractic Speaks Out: A Reply to Medical Propaganda, Bigotry and Ignorance*. Park Ridge, Ill.: Wilk Publishing Co., 1973.

M.B.H. Wilson. *Chiropractic: A Patient's Guide*. Rochester, Vt.: Thorsons Publishing Group, 1987.

Practice Guidelines for Straight Chiropractic: Proceedings of the International Straight Chiropractic Consensus Conference Chandler, Arizona 1992. Chandler, Ariz.: World Chiropractic Alliance, 1993.

Christian Science

R. Peel. *Mary Baker Eddy: The Years of Discovery*. New York: Holt, Rinehart and Winston, 1972.

Color breathing

L. Clark and Y. Martine. *Health, Youth, and Beauty through Color Breathing.* Berkeley, Cal.: Celestial Arts, 1976.

Color meditation (CM)

R. Buckland. *Practical Color Magick.* St. Paul, Minn.: Llewellyn Publications, 1984.

Color synergy

P. George and D. Lovett. *Color Synergy: How to Use the Power of Color, Affirmations, and Creative Visualizations to Transform Your Life.* New York: Simon & Schuster, 1990.

Concept therapy

T. Fleet. *The Cause of Disease.* San Antonio, Tex.: 1967.

_____ *Suggestive Therapy Applied: The Chiropractic Approach to the Treatment of Psychosomatic Disorders.* San Antonio, Tex.: Concept-Therapy Institute, 1977.

Cosmic vibrational healing

M. Smulkis and F. Rubenfeld. *Starlight Elixirs and Cosmic Vibrational Healing.* Saffron Walden, Essex, England: C.W. Daniel Co. Ltd., 1992.

Creative visualization

S. Gawain. *Creative Visualization.* New York: Bantam Books, 1982.

M.L. Rossman. *Healing Yourself: A Step-by-Step Program for Better Health through Imagery.* New York: Walker and Co., 1987.

Crystal therapy

P. Galde. *Crystal Healing: The Next Step.* St. Paul, Minn.: Llewellyn Publications, 1991.

P. Green and R. Hils. *Crystal Wisdom: A Beginner's Guide. Second Edition.* Atlanta: Blue Dolfyn Publishers, 1985.

Dayan Qigong

C. Zu and M. Yang. *Dayan Qigong.* Hong Kong: Peace Book Co. Ltd., 1986.

Diamond approach

A.H. Almaas. *Essence: The Diamond Approach to Inner Realization.* York Beach, Me.: Samuel Weiser, Inc., 1986.

Dreamwork

S. Kaplan-Williams. *The Elements of Dreamwork.* Rockport, Mass.: Element Inc., 1991.

Enneagram system

K.V. Hurley and T.E. Dobson. *What's My Type? Use the Enneagram System of Nine Personality Types to Discover Your Best Self.* San Francisco: HarperCollins Publishers, 1992.

D.R. Riso. *Enneagram Transformations: Releases and Affirmations for Healing Your Personality Type.* New York: Houghton Mifflin, 1993.

Eutony
G. Alexander. *Eutony: The Holistic Discovery of the Total Person.* Great Neck, N.Y.: Felix Morrow, 1985.

Gerson therapy
M. Gerson. *A Cancer Therapy: Results of Fifty Cases and the Cure of Advanced Cancer by Diet Therapy.* Bonita, Cal.: Gerson Institute, 1990.

Graphology, medical
M. de Surany. *Medical Graphology.* York Beach, Me.: Samuel Weiser, Inc., 1991.

Hatha yoga
R.L. Hittleman. *Richard Hittleman's Yoga 28 Day Exercise Plan.* New York: Bantam Books, 1973.
L. Lidell, Narayani, and G. Rabinovitch. *The Sivananda Companion to Yoga.* New York: Simon & Schuster, 1983.
Samskrti and Veda. *Hatha Yoga: Manual I. Second Edition.* Honesdale, Pa.: Himalayan International Institute of Yoga Science and Philosophy of the U.S.A., 1985.
W. Slater. *Hatha Yoga: A Simplified Course.* Wheaton, Ill.: Theosophical Publishing House, 1978.

Healing tao
*M. Chia and M. Chia. *Bone Marrow Nei Kung: Taoist Ways to Improve Your Health by Rejuvenating Your Bone Marrow and Blood.* Huntington, N.Y.: Healing Tao Books, 1989.

Hippocrates diet and health program
B.R. Clement: *Belief: All There Is.* West Palm Beach, Fla.: Hippocrates Publications, 1991.
_____ *Hippocrates Health Program: A Proven Guide to Healthful Living.* West Palm Beach, Fla.: Hippocrates Publications, 1989.
A. Wigmore. *The Hippocrates Diet and Health Program.* Wayne, N.J.: Avery Publishing Group Inc., 1984.

Homeopathy
H.L. Coulter. *Divided Legacy: The Conflict Between Homoeopathy and the American Medical Association.* Berkeley, Cal.: North Atlantic Books, 1982.
_____ *Homoeopathic Medicine.* St. Louis, Mo.: Formur, Inc., 1975.
K.A. Scott and L.A. McCourt. *Homoeopathy: The Potent Force of the Minimum Dose.* Wellingborough, Northamptonshire, Great Britain, 1982.
G. Vithoulkas. *Homeopathy: Medicine of the New Man.* New York: Simon & Schuster, 1987.
_____ *The Science of Homeopathy.* New York: Grove Press, Inc., 1981.

Imagineering
S. King. *Imagineering For Health: Self-Healing Through the Use of the Mind.* Wheaton, Ill.: Theosophical Publishing House, 1981.

Inner child therapy

J. Bradshaw. *Homecoming: Reclaiming and Championing Your Inner Child.* New York: Bantam Books, 1992.

Iridology

B. Jensen with K. Wills and M. Diogo. *Iridology Simplified. Fifth Edition.* Escondido, Cal.: Iridologists International, 1980.

Jungian psychology

C.G. Jung. *Modern Man in Search of a Soul.* New York: Harcourt Brace Jovanovich. First published in 1933.

―――― *The Undiscovered Self.* New York: Penguin Books, 1958.

Kriya yoga and Paramahansa Yogananda

L. Holt. Kriya yoga: Still alive and well in the New Age. *New Frontier,* October 1992, pp. 21–24.

G. Kriyananda. *Beginner's Guide to Meditation.* Chicago: Temple of Kriya Yoga, 1988.

P. Yogananda. *Autobiography of a Yogi.* Los Angeles: Self-Realization Fellowship, 1987.

―――― *How You Can Talk with God.* Los Angeles: Self-Realization Fellowship, 1957.

―――― *The Law of Success. Seventh Edition.* Los Angeles: Self-Realization Fellowship, 1980.

―――― *Metaphysical Meditations.* Los Angeles: Self-Realization Fellowship, 1964.

―――― *Scientific Healing Affirmations: Theory and Practice of Concentration.* Los Angeles: Self-Realization Fellowship, 1981.

Kulkarni naturopathy

V.M. Kulkarni. *Naturopathy: The Art of Drugless Healing. Second Edition.* Delhi, India: Sri Satguru Publications, 1986.

Lemonade diet

S. Burroughs. *Healing for the Age of Enlightenmentt. Fourth Edition.* Newcastle, Cal.: Stanley Burroughs, 1976.

Macfadden, Bernarr

J.L. Macfadden. *Barefoot in Eden: The Macfadden Plan for Health, Charm, and Long-Lasting Youth.* Englewood Cliffs, N.J.: Prentice-Hall, 1962.

Macrobiotics

H. Aihara. *Acid·and Alkaline. Fourth Edition.* Oroville, Cal.: George Ohsawa Macrobiotic Foundation, 1982.

D. Benedict. *Confessions of a Kamikaze Cowboy.* North Hollywood, Cal.: Newcastle Publishing Co., Inc., 1987.

V. Brown with S. Stayman. *Macrobiotic Miracle: How a Vermont Family Overcame Cancer.* New York: Japan Publications, Inc., 1984.

W. Dufty. *You Are All Sanpaku*. Secaucus, N.J.: Citadel Press, 1965.

E. Esko (ed.). *Doctors Look at Macrobiotics*. New York: Japan Publications, Inc., 1988.

_____ *Macrobiotics: Experience the Miracle of Life*. Brookline, Mass.: East West Health Books, 1985.

_____ *The Teachings of Michio Kushi: The Way of Life in the Age of Humanity*. Becket, Mass.: One Peaceful World Press, 1993.

J. Ineson. *The Way of Life: Macrobiotics and the Spirit of Christianity*. New York: Japan Publications, Inc., 1986.

*R.E. Kotzsch. *Macrobiotics: Yesterday and Today*. New York: Japan Publications, Inc., 1985.

M. Kushi. *The Book of Macrobiotics: The Universal Way of Health and Happiness*. Tokyo: Japan Publications, Inc., 1977.

_____ *Standard Macrobiotic Diet: A Guide to Balanced Eating with Endless Variety and Satisfaction*. Becket, Mass.: One Peaceful World Press, 1992.

_____ *Your Face Never Lies: An Introduction to Oriental Diagnosis*. Wayne, N.J.: Avery Publishing Group Inc., 1983.

M. Kushi and M.C. Cottrell with M.N. Mead. *AIDS, Macrobiotics, and Natural Immunity*. New York: Japan Publications, Inc., 1990.

M. Kushi with E. Esko. *The Macrobiotic Approach to Cancer: Towards Preventing and Controlling Cancer with Diet and Lifestyle*. Garden City Park, N.Y.: Avery Publishing Group Inc., 1991.

M. Kushi with A. Jack. *The Cancer Prevention Diet: Michio Kushi's Nutritional Blueprint for the Prevention and Relief of Disease*. New York: St. Martin's Press, 1983.

*T. Monte. *The Way of Hope: Michio Kushi's Anti-AIDS Program, The Drug-Free Way to Strengthen the Immune System through Macrobiotics*. New York: Warner Books, 1989.

G. Ohsawa. *Macrobiotics: An Invitation to Health and Happiness*. Oroville, Cal.: George Ohsawa Macrobiotic Foundation, 1971.

_____ *Philosophy of Oriental Medicine: Key to Your Personal Judging Ability*. *Eighth Edition*. Oroville, Cal.: George Ohsawa Macrobiotic Foundation, 1991. (Previously published as *The Book of Judgment*.)

*_____ *Zen Macrobiotics: The Philosophy of Oriental Medicine. Volume One*. Los Angeles: Ohsawa Foundation, Inc., 1965.

A.J. Sattilaro with T.J. Monte. *Living Well Naturally*. Boston: Houghton Mifflin, 1985.

*_____ *Recalled By Life*. New York: Avon Books, 1984.

Magical diet(s)

S. Cunningham. *The Magic in Food: Legends, Lore, and Spellwork*. St. Paul, Minn.: Llewellyn Publications, 1991.

Magical herbalism

S. Cunningham. *Magical Herbalism*. St. Paul, Minn.: Llewellyn Publications, 1983.

Meditation

R.M. Ballentine (ed.). *The Theory and Practice of Meditation. Second Edition.* Honesdale, Pa.: Himalayan International Institute of Yoga Science and Philosophy of the U.S.A., 1986.

A. Gardner. *Meditation: A Practical Study (with Exercises).* Wheaton, Ill.: Theosophical Publishing House, 1968.

Sri Ramakrishna Math (publisher). *Paths of Meditation: A Collection of Essays on Different Techniques of Meditation According to Different Faiths. Second Edition.* Madras, India: Sri Ramakrishna Math, 1984.

L.K. Misra. *The Art and Science of Meditation.* Glenview, Ill.: Himalayan International Institute of Yoga Science and Philosophy of the U.S.A., 1976.

Middle pillar meditation

M. Allen (ed.). *The Art of True Healing.* San Rafael, Cal.: New World Library, 1991.

Mucusless diet healing system

A. Ehret. *Mucusless Diet Healing System: A Scientific Method of Eating Your Way to Health.* New York: Benedict Lust Publications, 1970.

Natural Hygiene

H. Diamond and M. Diamond. *Fit For Life.* New York: Warner Books, 1987.

———— *Fit For Life II: Living Health.* New York: Warner Books, 1988.

T.C. Fry (ed.). *Guide to the Joyous Life. Volume I: The Greatest Health Discovery.* Pearsall, Tex.: Healthway Publications (c. 1975).

*T.C. Fry. *Program for Dynamic Health: An Introduction to Natural Hygiene, the Only True Health System.* Chicago: American Natural Hygiene Society, 1974.

D. Nelson. *Food Combining Simplified: How to Get the Most From Your Food.* 1985.

H.M. Shelton. *Food Combining Made Easy. Revised Edition.* San Antonio, Tex.: Willow Publishing, Inc., 1982.

———— *An Introduction to Natural Hygiene. Third Edition.* Mokelumne Hill, Cal.: Health Research, 1963.

———— *The Science and Fine Art of Fasting. Fifth Edition.* Chicago: Natural Hygiene Press, 1978.

———— *Superior Nutrition.* San Antonio, Tex.: Willow Publishing, Inc., 1987.

Nature cure

H. Lindlahr. *A Doctor's Views on Nature Care.* St. Catharines, Ont.: Provoker Press, 1972.

Naturopathy

P.O. Airola. *Are You Confused?* Sherwood, Ore.: Health Plus, 1972.

J.E. Pizzorno and M.T. Murray. *A Textbook of Natural Medicine. Volume I.* Seattle: John Bastyr College Publications, 1987.

R.F. Schmid. *Traditional Foods Are Your Best Medicine: Health and Longevity with the Animal, Sea, and Vegetable Foods of Our Ancestors.* New York: Ballantine Books, 1989.

R.N. Turner. *Naturopathic Medicine: Treating the Whole Person.* Wellingborough, Northamptonshire, England: Thorsons Publishers Ltd., 1990.

Nontraditional education
J. Bear. *College Degrees by Mail: 100 Good Schools That Offer Bachelor's, Master's, Doctorates, and Law Degrees by Home Study.* Berkeley, Cal.: Ten Speed Press, 1992.
_____ *Bear's Guide to Earning College Degrees Non-Traditionally. Eleventh Edition.* Benicia, Cal.: C & B Publishing, 1992.
_____ *Bear's Guide to Earning Non-Traditional College Degrees. Tenth Edition..* Berkeley, Cal.: Ten Speed Press, 1988.
C.D. Hayes. *Self-University.* Wasilla, Alas.: Autodidactic Press, 1989.
R.L.J. Walston and J. Bear. *Walston and Bear's Guide to Earning Religious Degrees Non-Traditionally.* Benicia, Cal.: C & B Publishing, 1993.

Numbers diet (Jean Simpson's numbers diet)
J. Simpson. *Jean Simpson's Numbers Diet.* New York: Crown Publishers, 1990.

Nutripathy
G.A. Martin. *Don't Eat the Yellow Snow: A New Holistic Approach to Health.* 1987.
_____ *Nutripathy . . . The Final Solution to Your Health Dilemma. Revised Tenth Edition.* Scottsdale, Ariz.: American College of Nutripathy (copyright 1978).

Nutritional herbology
M. Pedersen. *Nutritional Herbology.* Bountiful, Ut.: Pedersen Publishing, 1987.
_____ *Nutritional Herbology. Volume II: Herbal Combinations. Second Edition.* Spanish Fork, Ut.: Pedersen Publishing, 1990.

Occult medicine
J. Angelo. *Spiritual Healing: Energy Medicine for Today.* Rockport, Mass.: Element Inc., 1991.
B. Bloomfield. *The Mystique of Healing.* York Beach, Me.: Samuel Weiser, Inc., 1985.
F. Hartmann. *Occult Science in Medicine.* New York: Samuel Weiser, Inc., 1893.
G.W. Meek (ed.). *Healers and the Healing Process.* Wheaton, Ill.: Theosophical Publishing House, 1977.
C.N. Shealy with A.S. Freese. *Occult Medicine Can Save Your Life: A Modern Doctor Looks at Unconventional Healing.* Columbus, O.: Brindabella Books, 1985.

Organismic psychotherapy
M. Brown. *The Healing Touch: An Introduction to Organismic Psychotherapy.* Mendocino, Cal.: LifeRhythm, 1990.

Orgonomy
J. DeMeo. *The Orgone Accumulator Handbook: Construction Plans, Experimental Use and Protection Against Toxic Energy. Second Revised Edition.* El Cerrito, Cal.: Natural Energy Works, 1989.

Palmistry
*Cheiro the Palmist. *Comfort's Palmistry Guide*. Baltimore: I. & M. Ottenheimer (published around the turn of the century).

Plant alchemy (spagyrics)
M.M. Junius. *The Practical Handbook of Plant Alchemy: An Herbalist's Guide to Preparing Medicinal Essences, Tinctures, and Elixirs.* Rochester, Vt.: Healing Arts Press, 1993.

Polarity balancing
R. Gordon. *Your Healing Hands: The Polarity Experience.* Oakland, Cal.: Wingbow Press, 1984.

Pranic healing
*C.K. Sui. *Pranic Healing*. York Beach, Me.: Samuel Weiser, Inc., 1990.

"Psychology of evil"
M.S. Peck. *People of the Lie: The Hope for Healing Human Evil.* New York: Simon & Schuster, 1985.

_____ *The Road Less Traveled: A New Psychology of Love, Traditional Values and Spiritual Growth.* New York: Simon & Schuster, 1979.

_____ *Further Along The Road Less Traveled: The Unending Journey Toward Spiritual Growth. The Edited Lectures.* New York: Simon & Schuster, 1993.

Psychometric analysis
M.F. Long. *Psychometric Analysis.* Marina del Rey, Cal.: DeVorss & Co. (copyright 1959 by Huna Research Publications).

Radiance breathwork, radiance movement therapy, and radiance prenatal process
G. Hendricks and K. Hendricks. *Radiance! Breathwork, Movement and Body-Centered Psychotherapy.* Berkeley, Cal.: Wingbow Press, 1991.

Radiance technique
B. Ray. *The Official Handbook of The Radiance Technique.* Santa Monica, Cal.: American-International Reiki Association, Inc., 1987.

_____ *The 'Reiki' Factor in The Radiance Technique. Expanded Edition.* St. Petersburg, Fla.: Radiance Associates, 1992.

Radiesthesia
A. Mermet. *Principles and Practice of Radiesthesia: A Textbook for Practitioners and Students.* Shaftesbury, Dorset, Great Britain: Element Books Ltd., 1987.

Radionics
D.V. Tansley. *Radionic Healing: Is It for You?* Shaftesbury, Dorset, Great Britain: Element Books Ltd., 1988.

Rainbow diet
G. Cousens. *Spiritual Nutrition and The Rainbow Diet.* Boulder, Col.: Cassandra Press, 1986.

Reflexology
M. Carter. *Body Reflexology: Healing at Your Fingertips.* West Nyack, N.Y.: Parker Publishing Co., 1983.

Reiki
L. E. Arnold and S.K. Nevius. *The Reiki Handbook: A Manual for Students and Therapists of the Usui Shiko Ryoho System of Healing. Fourth Edition.* Harrisburg, Pa.: ParaScience International, 1992.
B. Baginski and S. Sharamon. *Reiki: Universal Life Energy.* Mendocino, Cal.: LifeRhythm, 1988.
A.L. Robertson. *Reiki.* St. Petersburg, Fla.: Omega Dawn Sanctuary of Healing Arts, 1989.
J. Stewart. *The Reiki Touch: A Reiki Handbook.* Houston: The Reiki Touch, Inc., 1990.

Reiki plus
D. G. Jarrell. *Reiki Plus Natural Healing: A Spiritual Guide to Reiki Plus. Fourth Edition.* 1991.

Schuessler biochemic system of medicine
G.W. Carey. *The Biochemic System of Medicine.* New Delhi, India: B. Jain Publishers Pvt. Ltd., 1991.

Self-healing (direct healing)
P. Ellsworth. *Direct Healing.* North Hollywood, Cal.: Newcastle Publishing Co., Inc., 1982.

Sotai
K. Hashimoto with Y. Kawakami. *Sotai: Balance and Health through Natural Movement.* Tokyo: Japan Publications, Inc., 1983.

Sufi healing
A.A.G. Moinuddin. *The Book of Sufi Healing. Revised and Updated Edition.* Rochester, Vt.: Inner Traditions International, Ltd., 1991.

Tai chi
Y. Tang. Scientific taijiquan. *Qi: The Journal of Traditional Eastern Health & Fitness,* Vol. 3, No. 1, Spring 1993, pp. 32–37.

Taoism
Tao: To Know and Not Be Knowing. San Francisco, Cal.: Chronicle Books, 1993.

Theosophy
*Alcyone (J. Krishnamurti). *At the Feet of the Master.* Wheaton, Ill.: Theosophical Publishing House, 1986.
A. Besant. *Death—and After?* Wheaton, Ill.: Theosophical Publishing House, 1893.
H.P. Blavatsky. *The Key to Theosophy. Simplified Edition.* Wheaton, Ill.: Theosophical Publishing House, 1953.

Theotherapy

P. Lemesurier. *The Healing of the Gods: The Magic of Symbols and the Practice of Theotherapy.* Shaftesbury, Dorset, Great Britain: Element Books Ltd., 1988.

Therapeutic touch

D. Krieger. *The Therapeutic Touch: How to Use Your Hands to Help or to Heal.* New York: Simon & Schuster, 1986.

Tibetan medicine

E. Finckh. *Studies in Tibetan Medicine.* Ithaca, N.Y.: Snow Lion Publications, 1988.

Tibetan pulsing healing

Shraddho. Tibetan pulsing healing. *Creations,* Vol. 7, No. 2, Spring (April/May) 1993, p. 9.

Trager mentastics

M. Trager with C. Guadagno-Hammond. *Trager Mentastics: Movement as a Way to Agelessness.* Barrytown, N.Y.: Station Hill Press, Inc., 1987.

Transcendental meditation (TM)

H.H. Bloomfield, M.P. Cain, and D.T. Jaffe, with R.B. Kory. *TM: Discovering Inner Energy and Overcoming Stress.* New York: Delacorte Press, 1975.

Twelve steps

J. Klaas. *The Twelve Steps to Happiness: A Handbook for All Twelve Steppers.* New York: Ballantine Books, 1990.

M. Beattie. *Codependents' Guide to the Twelve Steps.* New York: Simon & Schuster, 1992.

Urine therapy

B. Bartnett and M. Adelman. *The Miracles of Urine-Therapy.* Margate, Fla.: Lifestyle Institute, 1987.

Vibrational medicine

R. Gerber. Vibrational medicine. *Edges: New Planetary Patterns,* Vol. 2, No. 2, September 1989, pp. 14–17.

Vita flex

S. Burroughs. *Healing for the Age of Enlightenment. Fourth Edition.* Newcastle, Cal.: Stanley Burroughs, 1976.

Witchcraft

K. Paulsen. *The Complete Book of Magic and Witchcraft. Revised Edition.* New York: Penguin Books, 1980.

Zone therapy

A. Bergson and V. Tuchak. *Zone Therapy.* New York: Windsor Publishing Corp., 1974.

Reference Books

E.H. Ackerknecht. *A Short History of Medicine. Revised Edition.* Baltimore, Md.: Johns Hopkins University Press, 1982.

P. A. Angeles. *The HarperCollins Dictionary of Philosophy. Second Edition.* New York: HarperCollins Publishers, 1992.

A.L. Basham. *The Origins and Development of Classical Hinduism.* New York: Oxford University Press, 1991.

*E. Campbell and J.H. Brennan. *The Aquarian Guide to the New Age.* Wellingborough, Northamptonshire, England: Thorsons Publishing Group, 1990.

*R. Cavendish (ed.). *Encyclopedia of the Unexplained: Magic, Occultism and Parapsychology.* New York: Viking Penguin, 1989.

G. de Purucker. *Occult Glossary: A Compendium of Oriental and Theosophical Terms.* Pasadena, Cal.: Theosophical University Press (originally published in 1933).

*G. Dunwich. *The Concise Lexicon of the Occult.* New York: Carol Publishing Group, 1990.

I. Fischer-Schreiber, F. Ehrhard, and M.S. Diener. *The Shambhala Dictionary of Buddhism and Zen.* Boston: Shambhala Publications, 1991.

I. Fischer-Schreiber, F. Ehrhard, K. Friedrichs, and M.S. Diener. *The Encyclopedia of Eastern Philosophy and Religion.* Boston: Shambhala Publications, 1989.

A. Flew. *A Dictionary of Philosophy. Revised Second Edition.* New York: St. Martin's Press, 1984.

*R.E. Guiley. *Harper's Encyclopedia of Mystical and Paranormal Experience.* San Francisco: HarperCollins Publishers, 1991.

J.R. Hinnells. *A Handbook of Living Religions.* New York: Viking Penguin, 1985.

*S. Holroyd. *The Arkana Dictionary of New Perspectives.* New York: Viking Penguin, 1989.

*A. Jack (ed.). *The New Age Dictionary: A Guide to Planetary Family Consciousness. Revised and Enlarged Edition.* New York: Japan Publications, Inc., 1990.

D.M. Knipe. *Hinduism: Experiments in the Sacred.* San Francisco: HarperCollins Publishers, 1991.

G. MacGregor. *Dictionary of Religion and Philosophy.* New York: Paragon House, 1991.

Mysteries of Mind, Space & Time—The Unexplained. Westport, Ct.: H.S. Stuttman, Inc., 1992.

Mysteries of the Unknown: Ancient Wisdom and Secret Sects. Alexandria, Va.: Time-Life Books.

Mysteries of the Unknown: Eastern Mysteries. Alexandria, Va.: Time-Life Books.

Mysteries of the Unknown: Psychic Powers. Alexandria, Va.: Time-Life Books.

G. Parrinder (ed.). *World Religions From Ancient History to the Present.* New York: Facts On File Publications, 1984.

M. Random. *Japan: Strategy of the Unseen. A Guide for Westerners to the Mind of Modern Japan.* Wellingborough, Northamptonshire, England: Thorsons Publishing Group, 1987.

L. Spence. *The Encyclopedia of the Occult*. London: Bracken Books, 1988.
D. Watson. *The Dictionary of Mind and Spirit*. New York: Avon Books, 1992.
T.A. Wise. *The Hindu System of Medicine*. Delhi, India: Mittal Publications, 1986.
E. Wood. *Zen Dictionary*. Rutland, Vt.: Charles E. Tuttle Co., 1972.

Philosophy

*D. Kolak and R. Martin. *Wisdom without Answers: A Guide to the Experience of Philosophy*. Belmont, Cal.: Wadsworth Publishing Co., 1989.
*T. Nagel. *What Does It All Mean? A Very Short Introduction to Philosophy*. New York: Oxford University Press, 1987.
J. R. Searle. *Minds, Brains and Science*. Cambridge, Mass.: Harvard University Press, 1985.
*R. Taylor. *Metaphysics*. Englewood Cliffs, N.J.: Prentice-Hall, 1983.

Index

Mermet, Abbé Alexis, 218
Mesmer, Franciscus Antonius, 205
Metamorphic technique, 205
Metaphysical healing, 212
Metzner, Ralph, 55
Miasms, 106–107, 213
Microcosmic orbit meditation, 205
Middle pillar meditation, 205
Minarik, Richard, 31
Mind/body dualism, 24
Mind/body interactionism, 24
Mind-stuff theory, 24
Mitchell, S.W., 123
Monroe Institute, 191
Moody, Dr. Raymond, 71
Morrock, Richard, 32
Morter, Dr. M.T., Jr., 155–157
Morter HealthSystem, 155–157, 205
Moxabustion, 206
Moxibustion, 206
Moyers, Bill, 37, 38, 42–42
Mucusless diet healing system, 206
Muscle testing, 155, 227
Mystical Diets, 5
Mystical healing, 3
Mysticism, 24, 25
    proponent literature, 239

National Home Study Council, 90
National Institute of Medical Herbalists, 35
Natra-Bio, 105
"Natural healing," 98–99, 100, 107, 114, 232
Natural Health, 77
Natural Hygiene, 109–114, 206
Natural Law Party, 66–67
Natural laws, 97–99, 107
"Natural living," 109
Naturalism versus supernaturalism, 23–25
"Nature," 97
Nature cure, 206, 232
Nature's Sunshine Products, Inc., 208

Nature's Way Products, 105
Naturopathy, 101–104, 206
    HEW report on, 103
    involvement with homeopathy, 104–105
    Natural Hygiene, 109–114, 206
    schools, 104, 111
Nelson, Dr. Craig, 155
"Nerve energy," 152, 153
NETWORK, 206
Neural organization technique (NOT), 206
Neuro-linguistic programming (NLP), 195, 206–207
New Center for Wholistic Health Education and Research, 167
New Life Expo '91, 4
New York Actualism Center, 55, 165
New York Open Center, 119–120, 226
New York Wellness Body Center, 125
Newlife Expo, 4, 69, 119
Nightingale-Conant Corporation, 67, 172
Nirvana, 53
Nitikow, Dr. Dennis, 154
Nogier, Dr. P.F.M., 171
Nouthetic Counseling, 173
Numerology, 207–208
Nutripathy, 208
Nutritional herbology, 208

Object reading, 215
Ohashiatsu, 208
Ohsawa, George, 75, 77, 201
Okada, Kotama, 203
Oki-do, 208
OMEGA, 208
Omega Dawn Sanctuary of Healing Arts, 130
One Peaceful World, 76
Onomatomancy, 208
Oregon School of Herbal Studies, 35
Organic process therapy (OPT), 208–209